Birth Control on Main Street

Birth Control on Main Street

ORGANIZING CLINICS IN THE UNITED STATES, 1916–1939

Cathy Moran Hajo

University of Illinois Press
Urbana, Chicago, and Springfield

Manufactured in the United States of America
1 2 3 4 5 C P 5 4 3 2 1
This book is printed on acid-free paper.

Library of Congress Cataloging-in-Publication Data
Hajo, Cathy Moran.
Birth control on main street : organizing clinics in the United States, 1916–1939 / Cathy Moran Hajo. — Cloth & paper ed.
p. cm.
Includes bibliographical references and index.
ISBN 978-0-252-03536-4 (cloth : alk. paper)
ISBN 978-0-252-07725-8 (pbk. : alk. paper)
1. Birth control clinics—United States—History. 2. Birth control—United States—History. I. Title.
HQ766.5.U5H34 2010
363.9'60973—dc22 2009048718

To my daughter, Meg,
who can be the mother of
as many children as she wants

Contents

Acknowledgments

This book would not have been possible without the inspiration and guidance of Esther Katz, the editor and director of the Margaret Sanger Papers Project. It was she who encouraged me to pursue my studies while working as an editor at the Project, and she has been an enormous influence on my development as a historian, a researcher, and a documentary editor. Her support and friendship on this long journey have made each step easier. Peter C. Engelman, my colleague at the Project, is a wonderful sounding board and careful reader who helped me locate documents deep in the archives at Smith College that I would never have found on my own. I am also deeply grateful to Linda Gordon, who inspired me to develop my arguments more strongly and was generous with both advice and time when I was developing this work.

I owe a great debt to the scholars who went before me, often focusing on one locality or on a single aspect of the history of birth control. Their works were filled with insights that informed mine, particularly the work of Jessie Rodrique, Jimmy Elaine Meyer, Johanna Schoen, and Marianne Leung. A special thanks goes to Rosemarie Holz, whose writing on birth control clinics complemented and challenged mine. We met when both were in the early stages of our research, and while we could have easily become rivals, we instead became friends.

I must also acknowledge a debt to those who preserved the documents from which I wrote this history. To the birth control activists who recognized the value of their old files and the archivists and librarians who have taken such good care of them: thank you. While I mourn the many lost opportunities where records were destroyed, I value each available collection all the more. Special thanks go to: the Sophia Smith Collection at Smith College, the Francis A. Countway Library of Medicine at Harvard Medical School, and the Indiana Historical Society. In each institution, the archivists went out of their way to aid my research, and this history would be far less complete without their efforts. To Sherrill Redmon and Susan Boone at Smith, Jack Eckert at Countway, and Glenn McMullen at Indiana, thank you again.

I would like to thank the staff of the University of Illinois Press for their help in publishing this book and improving it along the way. Thanks to Joan Catapano, Alison Goebel, Louis Simon, and Angela Burton for bringing this book to fruition.

Life is not all about work and scholarship; the love and friendship of my friends and family were integral in enabling me to complete this work. Thanks to Brett George, Tom Frickanisce, and Dave and Ambra Pickett for their friendship over these many years. I want to thank my sister, Eileen Cosenza, her husband, James, and my nephews Kevin and Sean for the many hours we have spent together and the encouragement and love they have always shown. I would also like to thank my mother- and father-in-law, Farisa and Yadig Hajo, who welcomed me into their family with love and affection. My parents, Bob and Peggy Moran, have provided me with every conceivable help, starting when I was young and continuing to this day. Supportive, loving, and generous, they are simply the best parents a girl could have. Finally, my thanks and love go to Nabil, my wonderful husband, who has lived with birth control clinics, Margaret Sanger, and a distracted wife for far too long; and to my lovely daughter Meg, who makes it very hard to think about anything but her!

Abbreviations

ABCL	American Birth Control League
BCCRB	Birth Control Clinical Research Bureau
BCFA	Birth Control Federation of America
BCR	*Birth Control Review*
NCMH	National Committee on Maternal Health
CMHA	Cleveland Maternal Health Association
IBCL	Illinois Birth Control League
JOC	*Journal of Contraception*
NCFLBC	National Committee on Federal Legislation for Birth Control
PPFA	Planned Parenthood Federation of America

INTRODUCTION

The fight for reproductive rights was a critical event in the twentieth century, one that directly affected the lives of women and through them their husbands and children. Though less heralded than suffrage, in many ways it was a more sweeping reform, freeing many women from uncontrolled childbearing, which in turn allowed them to pursue other goals—equal rights, careers, or even the traditional roles of mother and wife. Feminist Crystal Eastman admitted: "Whether we are special followers of Alice Paul, or Ruth Law, or Ellen Key or Olive Schreiner, we must all be followers of Margaret Sanger. . . . We want this precious sex knowledge not just for ourselves, the conscious feminists; we want it for all the millions of unconscious feminists that swarm the earth—we want it for all women."[1] Birth control opened doors previously shuttered by family responsibilities, changing the role of sex in and outside of marriage. Eminently practical, birth control removed a major obstacle to a woman's emancipation, allowing her to plan her family in light of what she wanted to do with her life.

This book, focusing on the development of birth control clinics, takes a different look at the birth control movement in the first half of the twentieth century. While histories have been written about the fight for birth control, biographies dedicated to tracing the lives of its leaders, and local studies made of birth control activism in selected cities and states, birth control clinics have not received significant attention. Clinics were a crucial part of the birth control movement's drive to legitimize contraception, associating it not with immorality, but with maternal and infant welfare and public health. The clinic served many functions—a laboratory for testing the effectiveness and acceptability of new contraceptives, a place for activists to educate the public about birth control, and as tangible evidence that birth control was accepted and desired by the people the activists wanted to help. But first and foremost, it was a medical facility where patients were examined, prescribed contraceptives, and taught to use them. It was this practical function of the clinic that sets it apart from other birth control work and makes its story unique.

Under the leadership of Margaret Sanger, the birth control movement was a juggernaut that rapaciously collected any and all rationales defending a woman's right to choose. By the end of the 1930s, a gamut of arguments had been proffered. In the 1910s, anarchists called for birth control as a tool to deprive capitalists of fodder for their factories and wars. Socialists argued against the wealthy's monopoly on birth control knowledge, which they claimed kept the poor down. Feminists sought birth control as a means to emancipate women from the biological destiny that kept them tethered to the home. In the 1920s, rhetoric gradually shifted to the contention that birth control would improve public health, reduce infant and maternal mortality, and decrease the numbers of the unfit. By the mid-1930s, the emphasis shifted again, with activists arguing that government-sponsored contraceptives would reduce welfare burdens and help families deal with economic uncertainty. Activists combined these arguments when propagandizing for birth control, pushing one or more to the fore to win specific audiences and counter opposition. This makes it difficult to get a sense of what birth control activists really believed. Instead, one gets the sense that the movement was a hydra, whose many heads shouted different arguments, some contradicting others. Some claim that birth control activists fostered social control, eugenics, and the reduction of the numbers of the poor, immigrant, and nonwhite. Others see them as feminists who secured sexual freedom and wider opportunities for women; still others as maternalists, who worked to improve women and children's health without challenging the social and economic status quo. Because all of these arguments were used, sometimes in conjunction with one another, historians can find documents to back any and all of these interpretations.

My focus on the birth control clinic distinguishes between what activists *did* and what they *said.* We will look not only at their arguments, but at how they put those ideas into practice. Birth control clinics offer a unique microcosm of the larger movement that can reveal the weight that activists placed on specific issues. When activists argued that all women deserved the right to birth control knowledge, did they include unmarried women? When they claimed that the feebleminded should not propagate, who did they mean and who would diagnose this hazy condition? When they argued that the availability of birth control made women better mothers, how did they handle patients who wanted no children at all? The practical nature of clinic work offers an environment in which the historian can test the commitment of both activists and patients to the various threads of the movement's ideology, as it was the one place where activists interacted directly with those they were trying to help.

Chapter Overview

When I began my research I expected to find that most clinics behaved like smaller versions of Margaret Sanger's first doctor-run establishment. I thought to discern a clean line progressing from that model to the Planned Parenthood clinic of today. But the combination of private and public support for birth control that exists today was not the only way that contraceptive services could have proceeded. In the first two decades of clinic development there were several different models with no guarantee that any one would prevail. Local concerns, smoothed over in the descriptions of clinics made both by the national birth control movement and by most historians, turned out to be far more important to the success or failure of a clinic than the actions of organizations like the American Birth Control League or leaders like Margaret Sanger.

The first clinic in the United States was founded in 1916; prior to that, contraceptives and contraceptive information had been distributed through books, newspapers, magazine advertisements, and by word of mouth. The clinic was a hallmark of the modern birth control movement, relying on a physical site, medical staffing, and self-selected patients. Loosely adapted from the contraceptive clinics founded in the Netherlands, public health, and privately funded social welfare models, birth control clinics provided free or subsidized contraceptive advice to working-class women who lacked this knowledge.

Birth control clinics operated on two levels—as symbols of a national movement, but also as community-based centers. Unlike national work, local activists had to forge effective relationships with the doctors, social workers, politicians, religious leaders, and potential patients in their city. Working independently of medical and governmental health services, activists slowly convinced the public that health programs and hospitals should offer contraceptive services.[2] Clinic activists, the wives of business leaders, lawyers, and physicians, for the most part worked in a more cautious and cooperative manner than those who focused on education or legislation. Clinic activists learned that low-key lobbying among their wealthy peers and local medical societies were the keys to success. They rejected loud campaigns based on feminist or socioeconomic issues in favor of quiet and conservative lobbying for birth control on the basis of maternal health and economic responsibility. By the 1940s, these tactics had become the norm, as the national birth control movement became more conservative, relying on the participation of male professionals and physicians.

Chapter 1, "Birth Control Clinic Models," explains the lack of a single model for providing birth control services. Instead, activists developed "institutional" and "independent" clinics, each with strengths and weaknesses. Through the 1920s and 1930s both models were in play. While most activists preferred the idea of folding birth control into existing health institutions (hospitals and public health clinics), the most successful clinics in terms of patients treated were created and operated by independent birth control organizations. While activists knew that the independent clinic could never be sufficient to meet the nation's needs, it remained the backbone of the birth control movement well into the 1940s. Chapter 1 also traces the chronology of clinic development, from its beginnings in urban centers of the Northeast and Midwest, through the Depression years and the rapid spread to the South, smaller cities, and by 1939, to nearly every state in the Union.

Chapter 2, "Inside the Birth Control Clinic," explains what activists faced when providing clinical services. Activists had to weigh various birth control theories when setting policy and determining which services to include. A clinic's admission policies defined the kinds of women they wanted to treat. By comparing issues linked to birth control, such as abortion, sterilization, and unmarried patients, a clear picture of the self-imposed limitations of clinics emerges.

Chapter 3, "Clinic Activists," describes the women and men who devoted their time and money to this reform, laying out the tensions between them. Almost always founded and funded by lay women, power at the clinic remained in their hands throughout the decades. While the number of men participating in clinic work increased over the course of the 1920s and 1930s, lay women remained responsible for almost all day-to-day clinic operations.

Accusations of eugenics and racism plague birth control's legacy, and chapter 4, "Eugenics and Race at the Clinic," explores how these two important issues played out within clinic walls. It demonstrates that despite the hereditarian rhetoric favored by activists, the clinics based their work on environmental eugenics—the idea that it was not their genetic background, but available opportunities, that determined whether a person was "fit" or "unfit." Closely allied to views on eugenics were ideas about race. Birth control clinics were not places where white activists tried to reduce the populations of nonwhite patients. In fact, they were more likely to exclude admission to African Americans or segregate them into "black" clinics. While some activists argued for the establishment of African American clinics and hoped that African American activists would step up and create their own clinics, they offered little assistance to or acceptance of those who tried to do so.

Chapter 5, "The Clinic and Its Patients," shifts its focus to the women who attended the clinics. Without willing patients, clinics would not have been feasible, yet the motivations of patients, along with their views on birth control, differed from those of activists. By looking at who the patients were—their ages, income levels, reasons for attending the clinic, and their views on family and sex—we find them more discerning and active in their consumption of birth control than has been previously understood. Their views on marriage, gender roles, and sex, however, were more conservative and old-fashioned than those of the activists. When patients accepted the views on sex and marriage advanced by the clinic, they seem to have obtained more than just diaphragms and jelly—they were introduced to new ways of thinking about a woman's role in society.

The next two chapters situate the clinic in society, examining how local activists interacted with the state and the national birth control movement. In chapter 6, "Clinics and the Federal Government," I explore the Comstock Act's impact on clinic development. The law's focus on the mail limited its impact on clinics, as most information was provided in person. But by labeling birth control immoral and obscene, the Comstock Act had a major impact on efforts to secure institutional support. Neither the Children's Bureau nor the Public Health Service would support birth control, in large measure because of its dubious legal and moral status. While activists were able to secure limited local support for publicly funded birth control, they did not succeed in including contraceptive services in the Social Security or Sheppard-Towner Maternal Welfare programs.

Chapter 7, "Local Clinics and National Organizations," examines how local clinics negotiated the complex maze of birth control organizations in the 1930s, including the American Birth Control League, the National Committee for Federal Legislation on Birth Control, and the Birth Control Clinical Research Bureau, the last of which served not as a model for other clinics, but rather as a sort of über-clinic whose research and data analysis freed local clinics to concentrate on service. While clinic activists found the duplication of effort confusing, the competition for national supremacy helped to increase the creation of clinics. When the national groups merged at the end of the decade, the number of new clinics being founded began to decline.

Sources and Historiography

My interest in this topic came directly from my work with the Margaret Sanger Papers Project, which, though focused on the work of one activist, contains rich and deep documentation on the work of many clinics and local activists. I found Sanger's own clinic, the Birth Control Clinical Research Bureau (BCCRB), a fascinating enterprise, at once a charitable institution, research laboratory, public health clinic, and site for feminist awakening. I quickly noted, however, that most clinics were not nearly as elaborate or professional. Reading letters written by activists who wanted to start clinics, it became clear that there were many different ideas about how they should be organized. A point made by historian Ruth Crocker in another context proved instructive: "If Jane Addams and Hull House have dominated the historiography of the settlement movement, their prominence was no guarantee of typicality. Perhaps the typical settlement was a smaller, less distinguished Hull House, but then again it might have been altogether different. The point is not to discredit the achievements of the famous settlements. The point is that there was more to tell."[3] For the birth control clinic movement, Margaret Sanger and the BCCRB loom large over other activists and clinics, and have obscured our view of what else was happening. But while Sanger's leadership is integral to the story, there is, indeed, much more to tell. My goal is to focus on the development of birth control clinics as a national phenomenon, looking past the movement's rhetoric to uncover what the clinics were actually doing and how they worked.

The earliest sources describing birth control clinics were self-produced studies that presented descriptions and statistics, with a clear agenda—to prove the effectiveness and safety of birth control.[4] These books and articles provide demographic information on patients as well as some insight into their social and sexual lives. Though valuable as descriptive and quantitative sources, they are biased, never questioning the basic assumptions made by the clinics nor interrogating the data to find and explore anomalies. Because they are published and available, these studies have shaped the historiography of the clinic, as many historians look no further than the handful of reports documenting the BCCRB or Cleveland Maternal Health Association (CMHA).

To discover the range of clinic practices, I needed to broaden my sources. Luckily, descriptions of local leagues and clinic activities were published in birth control journals, such as the *Birth Control Review* (*BCR*) (1917–40) and the *Journal of Contraception* (*JOC*) (1935–39), as well as in newspapers and medical journals. These articles provide additional statistical data on the work of smaller clinics, and often supplied anecdotal stories about the clinic's founders, their patients, and their relations with local doctors, politicians, church leaders, and social workers.[5] Most clinic archives were not preserved and are not available to researchers. Where they have been archived, I have made use of board minutes, correspondence, newspaper articles, and various reports to flesh out the activities of the clinic and compare them with practices elsewhere. The records of national organizations and leaders have been particularly valuable for securing a broad representation of local reports.[6]

Clinics have not been a focus of the major histories on the fight for birth control. Though discussed in the context of the movement, most of these works try to analyze the work of national organizations, detailing the work of the American Birth Control League (ABCL), the struggle to legalize birth control, or the development of new contraceptive technologies. Clinics are part of those stories, but are never central to it. Books like Linda Gordon's *Woman's Body, Woman's Right* (revised as *The Moral Property of Women* in 2003), argue that the birth control movement gained momentum in the 1910s by linking arguments for birth control with calls for women's sexual and social freedom. As these aims were replaced by calls for improved maternal and infant health, race betterment, and economic planning in the 1920s, Gordon contends that the needs of families and society superseded those of individual women. The birth control clinic, the site where experts passed contraceptive information to patients, should be central to these contested changes. Gordon's influential take on the movement has become the base of later scholarship, but she looked broadly at the movement, focused on the relation of feminism to birth control, and did not study local activities or clinics. She argued that by the 1920s, the birth control movement was dominated by professionals, and the lay women who organized and funded the clinics had lost power.[7] While this holds for national organizations, the more we learn about local leagues and clinics the less it appears true. When one studies the records of a national organization, one assumes that the national organization directed grassroots activists. While the ABCL may have *wanted* to dominate local leagues and clinics, there is ample evidence that they had no such power. Histories of individual leagues and clinics often depict maverick clinics that ignored the national lead. As these "mavericks" multiply, the conclusion follows that the reach of the national league was far shorter than originally believed.

James Reed's *From Private Vice to Public Virtue: The Birth Control Movement and American Society since 1830* (1978) and Carole McCann's *Birth Control Politics in the United States, 1916–1945* (1994) both use the BCCRB to stand in for all clinics. In Reed's history, clinics form a small part of the story; instead, he focuses on the national movement's goals to popularize birth control in a medical setting and to develop new and better contraceptives. McCann looks more closely at clinics, seeing the drive to establish a nationwide chain of privately sponsored clinics as the chief goal of the American movement.[8] While she explored how this work demanded medical and eugenic allies as well as society women, she kept her focus on New York, Margaret Sanger, the ABCL, and the BCCRB. The thousands of local activists laboring across the country are assumed to be a loyal army spreading national policies under New York's direction.

Historians of local leagues paint a very different picture. They offer a brief overview of the national movement and short biography of Sanger and focus instead on who local activists were and what inspired them to start the clinic. In the rest of the story, if included at all, the national movement is rendered with broad strokes. Many make no distinction, for example, between the efforts of the BCCRB, the NCFLBC, and the ABCL in the 1930s, possibly because the local activists themselves did not always understand how or why the movement had split. These individual league and clinic studies often go overboard in asserting their clinic's unique independence from the national league, its rare emphasis on local politics and relations, and its generally more cautious approach to legal issues. Despite the efforts of the national movement to standardize clinical practice and reporting, local activists usually only adopted the parts of the national program that suited them.[9] Simone Caron's recent *Who Chooses?* tells a national story about the development of contraception, abortion, and sterilization in America, ending each chapter with a contrast with the experiences of the Rhode Island Birth Control League. Caron, as others before her, pits a feisty woman-centered clinic/league against a soulless and overly bureaucratized ABCL, which pushed an agenda limiting women's control over their lives and kowtowed to the medical profession.[10] Most of these works provide a detailed study of the clinic within the larger life of a city or state; others focus on issues of race, eugenics, or government control of fertility. Some situate their "exceptional" clinic within the national movement, but most use only a handful of secondary sources to paint a fairly superficial picture of the relationship between the two. As more and more "exceptional" clinics emerged, it became clear that it was the BCCRB that was unique, and that the real story of birth control clinics would come only by aggregating the stories of many maverick clinics.

Only a few historians have compared the experience of many clinics and leagues and they usually focus on a specific theme. Rosemarie Petra Holz's "The Birth Control Clinic in America: Life Within, Life Without, 1923–1972" (2002), takes the broadest look, focusing on the relationship of the clinic to the contraceptive marketplace. With a focus on Chicago-based clinics, Holz situates nonprofit clinics as just one of many choices patients had to obtain contraceptives. Her take on nonprofit clinics is that activists sought to monopolize the methods of birth control in order to win the support of the medical profession. She provides a unique juxtaposition between the work of these activists and that of contraceptive manufacturers and for-profit clinics, finding that activists defined respectability as medically controlled contraceptives in a charity clinical setting.[11]

A Short Trip through the History of Birth Control

For those unfamiliar with the general history of the birth control movement, including the activities of leaders like Margaret Sanger and of the various birth control organizations that flourished in the twentieth century, this overview will help to ground the analysis of clinics that follows.[12]

The Prehistory of Birth Control: The Nineteenth Century to 1916

There was no organized birth control movement in the early nineteenth century. In both Britain and America, public discussion of contraceptives only really began in the 1830s, in reaction to the economic theories of Rev. Thomas Malthus. By mid century, marital fertility, especially among the middle class, began a precipitous decline as industrialization brought with it new ideas about the optimum size of the family. But contraceptives were suspect, and those that promoted them were not usually doctors or feminists, but individuals seeking to make a profit.[13] The most common methods were simple practices such as douching, withdrawal, and abstinence, which usually required the cooperation of husbands with their wives.[14] As more people began trying to limit their families, a burgeoning market in euphemistically named "feminine hygiene" products sprang up to cater to the growing desires of middle-class whites.[15]

In the nineteenth century, written texts—books, pamphlets, and advertisements—were the most common means of obtaining contraceptive information.[16] Among the authors who spread the word in the United States were Robert Dale Owen, Charles Knowlton, and Frederick Hollick. These men were not regularly trained physicians; they were free thinkers or irregular physicians. Organized medicine, engaged in the process of professionalizing, scorned contraception as controversial and sordid, and allied with purity reformers to condemn contraceptive practices as immoral.[17] In 1873, the United States passed the Comstock Act, which forbade the use of the mails for the distribution of immoral articles, specifically including information and devices for contraception and abortion. Over the next ten years, the federal statute was copied by most states, prohibiting the spread of contraceptive advice, generally making no exemption for licensed doctors, druggists, or nurses. Thus the first chapter of the birth control movement's history was entwined with the free speech movement. Its defenders came from the fringes—free thinkers, anarchists, and sex radicals. Neither physicians nor feminists challenged the association of birth control with immorality.[18]

The impact of the Comstock Law upon contraceptive practice was mixed. Rather than stopping abortions and contraception, it drove the practices underground. While devices and advice books could still be had by the persistent, the quality of these materials declined as reprints of older texts were published with specific contraceptive information cut out to pass the censor's scrutiny. This left information less reliable, less accurate, and often badly written.[19]

It was not in America, but in the Netherlands, that the world's first birth control clinic was founded, in 1882. The clinic was operated by Aletta Jacobs, Holland's first female physician, a feminist, socialist, and suffragist, with an interest in preventing unwanted pregnancies. Jacobs's concern for the poor was sparked during her medical education and she began providing poor women with infant and child care education. At her Amsterdam clinic, Jacobs prescribed diaphragms for her patients, who returned for monthly follow-up visits until the doctor was assured that the method was working. Jacobs's clinic aroused the ire of the medical community, especially obstetricians, who feared that her charity clinic competed unfairly with their practices. Jacobs did not agree, recalling, "I felt that the longing to have a child is so strong in most normal women that only for the most serious reasons would they choose to avoid motherhood."[20] She kept the clinic open until her retirement twelve years later. Dr. Johannes Rutgers, a socialist and founding member of the Dutch Neo-Malthusian League, continued Jacobs's work. Unlike Jacobs, who thought that clinics should be run by doctors, Rutgers was eager to work with lay women. He opened free clinics for working-class women, training midwives and former patients, whom he called "lay-nurses," in the basics of the female reproductive system and the diaphragm. Then they were sent back to their neighborhoods to aid others.[21] For almost forty years, Malthusians and others in Europe watched the Dutch clinic experiment, but did not start their own. It was not until 1916 that another activist, American nurse Margaret Sanger, opened the next clinic.

Born to working-class Irish immigrant parents in 1879, Margaret Sanger had already brushed against the Comstock Act in 1913, when she battled censors who banned her frank discussion of venereal disease in the socialist paper, the *New York Call.* It was her 1914 journal, *The Woman Rebel,* however, that put her on the map. Sanger and her editorial staff coined the new term, "birth control," and she linked it to class warfare, feminism, and free love.[22] Sanger's political thinking was influenced by Emma Goldman when she started her campaign, but she was also deeply affected by the premature death of her mother after bearing eleven children. She quickly developed her own unique style and single-minded focus, which would launch the reproductive rights movement.[23]

In November 1914 she arrived in England, fleeing Comstock Act prosecution. There she met a wide range of British neo-Malthusians, from sexual theorists Havelock Ellis and Edward Carpenter, to socialist-feminist Stella Browne, and the politically conservative Drysdales. Both Ellis and the Drysdales advised

Sanger to visit the Dutch clinics. This brief exile was a watershed for Sanger, changing the direction of her thinking. During those months she fused the radicalism of the American movement, the theory of the British movement, and the practicality of the Dutch into something new and exciting. A nurse by training, though she never completed her degree, Sanger spent two weeks with Rutgers, learning to fit diaphragms and observing his clinics. Looking back on her experience, she later claimed that it was then that she realized that birth control had to involve medical staff, because the diaphragm method required a careful medical examination. It seems clear that Sanger initially thought that she could copy the Dutch clinic in America, because shortly after her return in October 1915, she announced plans to open a birth control clinic in the Lower East Side of New York City. As a nurse, a socialist, and a working-class radical, the Rutgers clinic model must have seemed attractive to Sanger. Having researched contraceptive methods to write *Family Limitation* (1914), *English Methods of Birth Control*, *Dutch Methods of Birth Control*, and *Magnetation Methods of Birth Control* (all 1915), she considered herself expert enough to operate her own clinic.

After a nationwide birth control lecture tour in 1916, Sanger opened her version of a Rutgers-style clinic on October 16, 1916. It was located in the immigrant neighborhood of Brownsville, Brooklyn. She was joined by her sister, Ethel Higgins Byrne (a registered nurse), and Fania Mindell (an interpreter). The Brownsville clinic was a direct challenge to New York State's obscenity law, which prohibited providing information on contraception or telling people where they could obtain such information. Sanger and her co-workers did not have a doctor on staff, nor did they actually examine and fit patients. Instead they explained how conception worked, advised women to purchase a specific diaphragm and contraceptive jelly at a nearby drugstore, and sold Sanger's pamphlets and books.[24] Sanger garnered headlines, goading the authorities in the press. "The police are hunting my clinic today," she crowed six days after opening it, "They can't find it. If they should, they can't hurt it. It is an oral clinic and the law says nothing about not spreading birth control information orally. If they do try to interfere I am legally prepared to carry a hard and bitter fight to the highest tribunal in the land, with the best legal talent there is."[25] The police found her clinic, raided it, and closed it down. Sanger, Byrne, and Mindell were arrested, tried, and convicted of violating the law. Sanger and Byrne were sentenced to thirty days in prison. On appeal, the New York State Supreme Court upheld Sanger's conviction but interpreted the law so that if she had employed a physician and treated women for medical reasons, she would not have violated the law.[26] Satisfied for the moment with this limited victory, Sanger based a clinic movement upon it.

Boosting Leagues and Clinics, 1916–29

In the immediate aftermath of the Brownsville clinic, the United States' entry into World War I disrupted any plans Sanger might have had to re-open her clinic. The fledgling birth control movement, mostly populated with socialists, radicals, and free love advocates, collapsed during the war. In 1917, Sanger started the *BCR*, a monthly journal of arguments for birth control and news about the doings of activists in the United States and abroad. She wrote *Woman and the New Race* (1920), a feminist argument for contraception that called on newly emancipated women to seize the issue and make it their own.

In 1921, Sanger founded the American Birth Control League (ABCL), a New York-based organization of mostly upper-class women, in order to educate the public and the medical profession about the benefits of birth control, to provide information about organizing state and city leagues, to promote the creation of clinics, and to lobby for the repeal of state and federal laws that lumped birth control with obscenity. In its early years, the ABCL served mostly as a support staff for Sanger's lectures, sponsoring the *BCR* and slowly gathering state affiliates and the support of a medical committee. New York state law did not permit the league to operate a medical clinic, but it appears that Sanger continued providing contraceptive advice privately, out of the league's offices on Fifth Avenue. In 1923 she opened the Clinical Research Bureau (BCCRB), in offices across the hall from the ABCL, the first legal clinic to operate in the United States.[27] The BCCRB was doctor-staffed, followed the letter of the law, and used its experiences to convince physicians, lawmakers, and the general public that birth control was safe, wanted, and effective.

Sanger saw the BCCRB as a model for other clinics and traveled around the country to speak on the clinic's work and to attract followers. In the next six years, almost thirty clinics were founded, mostly in large cities in the East and Midwest. As more clinics and leagues got underway, the ABCL changed, starting to undertake work independently of Sanger and catering to the needs of the new leagues and clinics. They tried and failed to effect legislative change in Washington and in New York and several neighboring states in the mid-1920s, but succeeded in holding regional conferences that brought women together and inspired them. In these years, Sanger initiated an international birth control movement and in 1925 hosted, through the ABCL, the first international gathering on birth control in the United States; she also spearheaded the organization of the World Population Conference in Geneva in 1927.[28]

Sanger's interest in international organization meant that she was often away from New York, particularly in 1926 and 1927. While she was away, the ABCL became used to doing things its own way. The women who ran the league were more conservative than Sanger and had backgrounds in social work and charitable organizing. They tried to turn the ABCL into a more efficient organization, and one far less accommodating to their law-defying, headline-grabbing president. When Sanger returned to New York in 1927, she was at odds with the ABCL's Executive Committee, headed by Eleanor Dwight Jones, over the new mission and tactics. After a few months of acrimony, Sanger surprised most observers by resigning in 1928. The divorce was kept quiet, but was not amicable, as the two fought over the "children" (in this case the BCCRB and the *BCR*). In the end, Sanger took the clinic and the ABCL kept the journal.[29]

By the end of the 1920s, Sanger was the most famous birth control activist in the country, possibly even the world. Known for her work with the clinic and the international movement, she added a new interest in 1929, agreeing to chair a committee dedicated to overturn the Comstock Act. Though the committee was originally conceived of as a part of the ABCL, Sanger's selection as chairwoman meant that it would become an autonomous organization, and in only a few years it would rival and perhaps surpass the ABCL.

Competition Is Good for Birth Control, 1930–37

The National Committee on Federal Legislation for Birth Control (NCFLBC), Sanger's lobbying league, was organized differently than the ABCL. Sanger adopted a geographic model, appointing chairs in each state and middle managers in charge of specific regions of the country, but policy and legislative tactics came from her central office. Because the NCFLBC was chiefly a lobbying organization, albeit with an educational component, it did not initially set up clinics or leagues. But it did send out field workers to organize support for its bills, and that brought the committee in touch with interested activists who, after hearing presentations on the NCFLBC's proposed bill, formed birth control leagues and sometimes clinics. While the NCFLBC was delighted with its impact, it was the BCCRB that Sanger had assist activists with establishing and managing clinics, providing them with information, supplies, and models of procedure.

Without Margaret Sanger's high profile, fund-raising clout, and the BCCRB, the ABCL was decidedly a weakened organization. Sanger's resignation, coinciding with the stock market crash, cost the ABCL dearly. Chronically short of funds, the ABCL treaded water for several years, focusing on publishing the *BCR* and producing educational materials.[30] Sending ABCL field workers to areas that were not organized for birth control or that needed help establishing or expanding their movement resulted in a steady increase in the numbers of clinics and leagues, all invited to affiliate with the national organization. The ABCL hoped to fund its field work and operating costs by collecting a percent of the donations taken in by its affiliates.[31] But for this to work they needed affiliation to carry weight with either patients or the medical profession, or else the new clinics and leagues would refuse to contribute.

As Sanger grabbed the headlines in the high-profile world of political lobbying, she expanded the BCCRB's responsibilities. As the ABCL methodically pursued the creation of state affiliates and clinics, they ran across NCFLBC and BCCRB field workers competing for the attention of local activists. Though Sanger and the ABCL unofficially divided birth control work between them—with the ABCL taking most of the educational efforts and organizing state leagues, Sanger's NCFLBC working on legislative efforts, and the BCCRB providing technical advice to clinics—in practice the lines became very blurry, especially to the field workers on the ground. After 1935, when both the ABCL and BCCRB prioritized the founding of clinics, numbers grew rapidly. Both organizations were bent on winning local endorsements, promising funds, supplies, advice, and training. The more the turf battles heated up, the more aid local activists were given. While the duplication of effort was wasteful, the competition between the two organizations made this a time of rapid expansion for clinics.

The Depression both harmed and helped the birth control movement. Activists found it more difficult to raise the funds needed to operate clinics and leagues, but the economic malaise helped to win over public opinion. The reality of the high costs of welfare, combined with an uncertain job market, made birth control seem a viable choice, certainly for those under- or unemployed, but also for middle-class families who wanted to keep up their pre-Depression quality of life.[32]

The center of activism in the 1930s was Sanger's legislative work. The NCFLBC drew up bills each year, secured sponsors, and then watched them die in committee, or in one instance be passed but then recalled on a technicality.[33] The Catholic Church increased its opposition to birth control, fighting not only legislative efforts, but also the movement's attempts to win the support of the American Medical Association and other influential groups. The ABCL continued fostering the creation of state leagues, aiding them in establishing city leagues that would operate clinics.[34]

In 1937, Sanger's team won a judicial ruling in *U.S. v. One Package*, which essentially won for doctors the right to use the mails to send and receive contraceptive information and devices. This made the NCFLBC's mission to rewrite the law moot. Sanger had the choice to either continue working to extend exemptions to the federal law (to include economic and social causes), to work to repeal state bans, or to declare victory. Worn out by the years of lobbying and raising funds in Depression-era America, Sanger chose the latter, disbanding the NCFLBC in a showy celebration of victory.[35] Sanger moved most of the NCFLBC's workers, field work programs, and contacts to the BCCRB. The BCCRB began to shift to become a broader based movement, involved with more than just clinical practice and testing contraceptives. Field work programs were offered, helping activists to open clinics, test new contraceptives, and organize public support for birth control. The BCCRB expanded its educational work and started a new national magazine and a program for certifying clinics. As the ABCL and BCCRB bickered over who had the right to organize certain states or whose affiliation program was more useful or prestigious, the squabbling and duplicated effort became obviously counterproductive. Analyses done for the ABCL by public relations experts found that the movement was wasteful, which drove away potential funders. It also acknowledged "the Sanger problem"—the fact that Margaret Sanger was a superior fund-raiser and the public face of the birth control movement. Any birth control organization that wanted to be taken seriously needed her backing.[36]

Coming Together Again: 1938–39

These battles cost the birth control movement. Field work programs were expensive, as was the burgeoning staff needed to oversee them. Resources to fund this kind of work were hard to come by. The sniping and pettiness also put off philanthropists who might have supported a unified movement. Sanger, though a thorn to the ABCL leadership, had to be a part of any merger, because her name brought recognition, legitimacy, and fund-raising skills. However, few ABCL officers could abide her imperious management style.

Distrust between the staffs of the BCCRB and the ABCL hampered negotiations, which failed in 1937 amidst mutual accusations of noncooperation.[37] By July 1938, a new and more positive spirit was born, largely created by Sanger's decision to step back from the movement into semi-retirement.[38] Tired after years of campaigning, she now spent most of her time in Tucson, far from the squabbles and petty politics of the league and bureau. As she wrote to Robert Dickinson after the merger was finalized, "For my part I made up my mind some months ago that if the merger was to take place I was going to give it my unqualified faith and support. I wanted it so much I was willing to make small compromises as to personnel and method."[39]

The new organization, the Birth Control Federation of America (BCFA), formed in January 1939, remade the movement on the ABCL's terms. Sanger yielded to the entreaties of the ABCL's organizers, who painted a picture of a stronger, more mainstream organization that would push to include birth control in public health programs. Sanger's retirement to Tucson took her away from daily interaction with both the clinic and the national leaders, and Hannah Stone's untimely death in 1941 left the BCCRB without an effective medical director.[40] Sanger allowed the BCFA activists to use her name for publicity and fund-raising, but avoided the efforts of her friends and colleagues to pull her back into a leadership role. Happy at first to be the grande dame of the movement, the honeymoon did not last, and Sanger became increasingly critical of and withdrawn from the efforts of the BCFA (after 1942 known as the Planned Parenthood Federation of America). She eventually threw herself into the postwar international birth control movement, helping to found the International Planned Parenthood Federation and working to develop an oral contraceptive. But that is a story for another day.[41]

ONE

Birth Control Clinic Models

The birth control clinic did not rise, fully formed, from Margaret Sanger's imagination. The Brownsville clinic, modeled on the contraceptive services Sanger had seen in the Netherlands, was not a viable American model given the restrictive laws and medical opposition. For the next seven years, Sanger gathered mainstream support for birth control, founding the ABCL in 1921 and working to popularize health and welfare rationales for contraception. Sanger next founded the Birth Control Clinical Research Bureau (BCCRB) in 1923, a doctor-run clinic based on a dispensary model. While this lay-driven "independent" clinic became the most influential model for providing birth control in the 1920s and 1930s, it was never planned as a permanent solution. Birth control activists like Sanger wanted hospitals or the government to take responsibility for the service, and though they created independent clinics in the interim, they never abandoned this goal. Despite some success, institutional clinics never replaced independent clinics, either numerically or in patients served. By the end of the 1930s, no one type of clinic predominated; instead the national birth control movement presided over a loosely linked patchwork of clinics that only partially covered the nation's cities and did not reach its rural depths. This chapter investigates the creation of these clinic models, looking at the strengths and weaknesses of each, and why none were suited to provide cohesive nationwide service.[1]

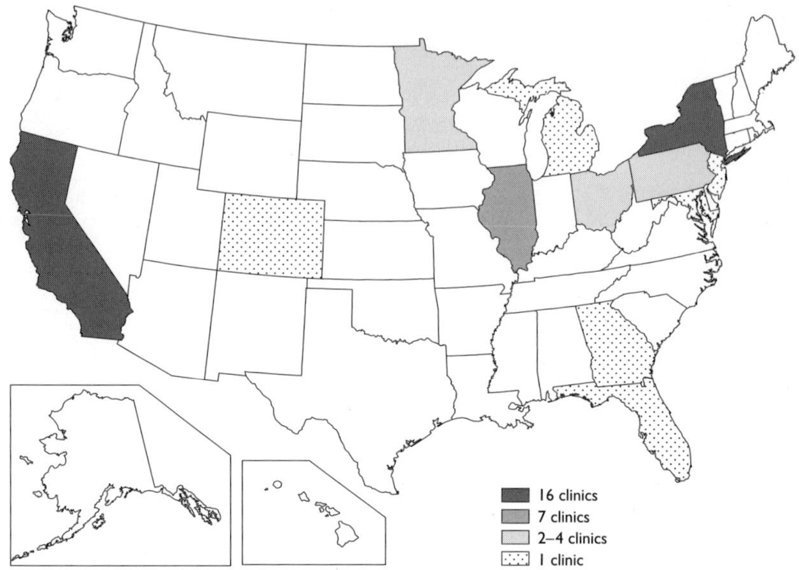

Map 1. Clinics, 1916–1929

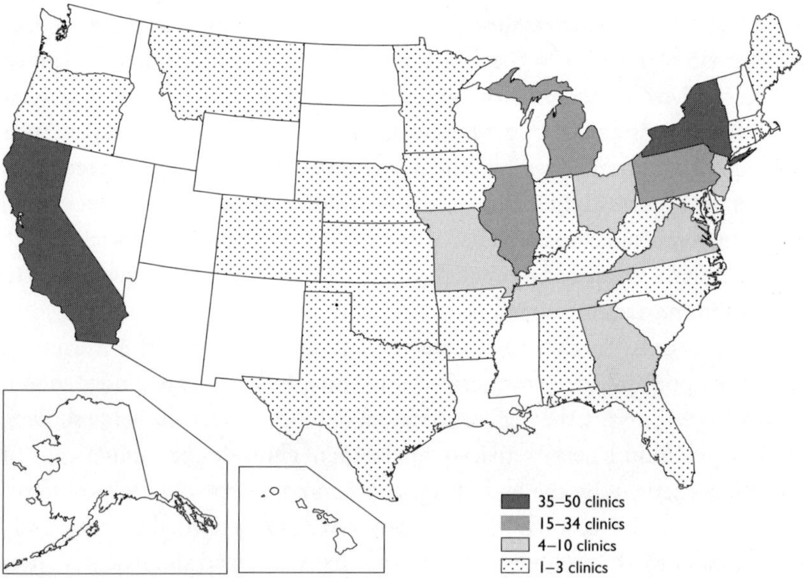

Map 2. Clinics, 1916–1934

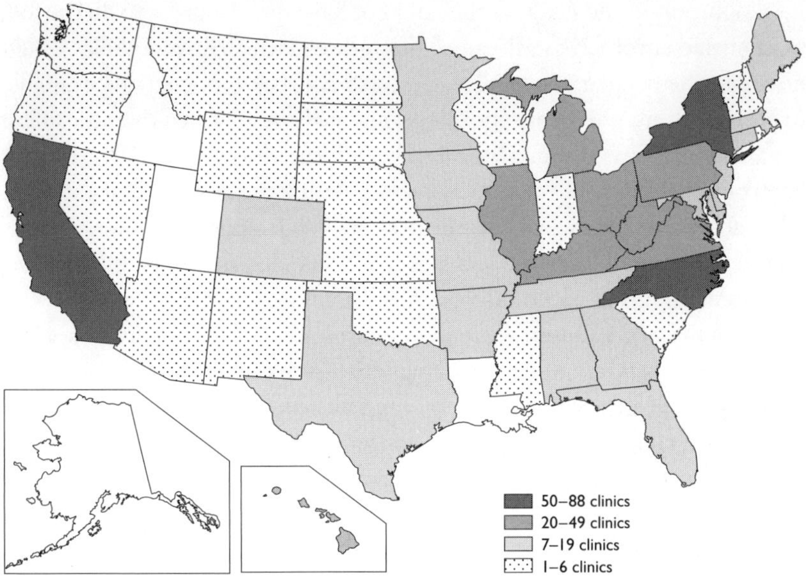

Map 3. Clinics, 1916–1939

Between 1916 and 1939, more than 650 clinics were founded in the United States. Some remain in operation today, while far more closed after a few months or years. Only thirty-nine clinics were created by 1929, but these pioneers inspired other activists to follow suit. In the first half of the 1930s, new clinic formation increased more rapidly, from a total of 55 in 1930 to 232 in 1935. But the most rapid expansion occurred between 1936 and 1938, fueled both by the work of national birth control leagues and the extension of birth control into state public health services. In 1936 alone, more than a hundred new clinics were founded, and increases continued until 1939. By 1940 there were 507 clinics operating in the United States.

Almost from the start, birth control activists agonized over whether they should create and fund freestanding clinics or work with the public and private health and welfare system to incorporate birth control into existing services. Independent and institutional clinics had strengths and drawbacks, so choosing between them was difficult. Independently operated clinics required more time and money, but were more popular with patients and easier for activists to control. Activists knew, however, that such clinics could never meet the nation's need.

Cognizant of the fact that they did not have the resources to do the job, most birth control activists dreamed of a future in which private clinics would no longer be needed. They expected birth control to one day be available to all via private physicians, hospitals, and government health and welfare departments. They thought the public, educated to the benefits of birth control, would demand contraceptives to tailor the size of their families. They accepted that they needed to start the ball rolling by founding clinics that demonstrated effectiveness and need. Aided by activists, model clinics sprang up in the 1920s in New York hospitals, California public health departments, and Chicago settlement houses. But activists found that when contraceptive services were added to existing programs at these institutions, the clinic itself was changed. They found institutional clinics less committed to birth control than the ones founded by birth control organizations. Institutions were highly selective in the patients they admitted and shied from advertising their service. Activists also found that many institutional clinics lacked a patient-friendly atmosphere. While institutional clinics made sense economically, practically they were attractive neither to the hosts nor to the patients.

Birth control activists grappled with the dilemma of choosing between establishing independent clinics and trying to gain access to the larger health care system, which risked some or all control over the work. Even as they continued founding clinics, lay activists tried to convince doctors and government officials to get into the contraceptive business, inviting them to join the national birth control movement and the advisory boards of local clinics. By the late 1930s, the ABCL and BCFA were encouraging the creation of institutional clinics at the expense of independent clinics, deriding the latter as old-fashioned and ineffective.[2]

But the rush to discard the independent clinic was premature. Institutional clinics, especially those located in hospitals, foundered on a lack of commitment. In 1930, 60 percent of all clinics were based in institutions (33 percent in hospitals, 18 percent government-sponsored, and 8 percent in settlements), with 40 percent of clinics independently run. Despite the efforts of the national movement to create more institutional clinics, in the 1930s the percentage of institutional clinics shrank steadily, to a low of 37 percent. When it began inching up again in 1939, it was due to the sudden creation of sixty-two public health clinics in North Carolina, a somewhat misleading statistic, as each of these clinics treated an average of only ten patients a year.[3] By 1939, only 18 percent of clinics were located in hospitals, with 58 percent in independent settings. By the end of the 1930s, it was clear that despite all the efforts of national activists, institutions would not supplant independent clinics.

The Independent Clinic

The majority of birth control clinics founded in the United States were "independent," meaning they were founded and operated by birth control leagues (see table 1). These leagues secured space, staff, and materials, advertised for patients, and kept records of treatments and results. Of the 654 clinics I have identified, 379 were independently run (58 percent). In terms of patient care they were even more influential. While the busiest hospital or government-run clinic might see 2,600 patients in a year, the top independent clinic, the BCCRB, saw that many in two or three months. In fact, several large independent clinics treated more patients each year than all institutional clinics combined. Independent clinics were also responsible for contraceptive research, training doctors, nurses, and medical students in the techniques of contraception, marriage counseling, and providing referrals to medical and welfare clinics for patients who suffered from other conditions. After years of propaganda, it was the independent clinic that most people pictured when they heard the words "birth control clinic," a woman-centered environment where mothers could find compassion and expert help. In Margaret Sanger's idealistic view, independent clinics offered something different from other clinics, providing "an atmosphere of welcome, of kindness, of understanding, where the women may come and tell us their troubles and be received with understanding and not with suspicion or derision."[4] Activists popularized this description to overcome the distrust that many women had for hospitals, the discomfort that they felt talking with doctors about sex matters, and the resentment they felt toward "do-gooders" who treated them shabbily in charity situations. But there was also truth to the idea that independent clinics were more patient centered.

Both of Sanger's clinics, the Brownsville clinic and the BCCRB, were independent. Brownsville, located in a store front, was the humbler of the two. Staffed by Sanger, a nurse, and an interpreter, the clinic was stark and ill-equipped, relying mostly on verbal instruction and referrals to local drugstores for diaphragms. Crowded with more than 480 patients in its ten-day lifespan, the Brownsville clinic demonstrated successfully its patients' need. Sanger likely expected it would be quickly closed and did not intend it to serve as a model for other clinics. Though she claimed, "In less than a year, there

Table 1. Clinics in Operation Each Year by Type (1916–40). For a complete listing of clinics, see http://www.press.uillinois.edu/books/hajo/appendix.php

Year	All	Independent Clinics		Institutional Clinics							
				Total		Hospitals		Government		Settlement	
Count		Count/%All		Count/%All		Count/%All		Count/%All		Count/%All	
1916	2	2	100	0	0	0	0	0	0	0	0
1923	4	2	50	2	50	2	50	0	0	0	0
1924	5	3	60	2	40	2	40	0	0	0	0
1925	9	6	67	3	33	3	33	0	0	0	0
1926	16	7	44	9	56	8	50	0	0	1	6
1927	23	10	43	13	57	7	30	3	13	3	13
1928	28	13	46	15	54	6	21	6	21	3	11
1929	42	19	45	23	55	10	24	10	24	3	7
1930	60	24	40	36	60	20	33	11	18	5	8
1931	101	43	43	58	57	35	35	14	14	9	9
1932	135	65	48	70	52	43	32	16	12	11	8
1933	172	89	52	83	48	50	29	19	11	14	8
1934	187	105	56	82	44	50	27	15	8	17	9
1935	249	157	63	92	37	55	22	20	8	17	7
1936	353	224	63	129	37	76	22	28	8	25	7
1937	431	273	63	158	37	85	20	48	11	25	6
1938	463	292	63	171	37	82	18	67	14	22	5
1939	428	249	58	179	42	78	18	78	18	23	5
1940	507	267	53	240	47	83	16	137	27	20	4

Sources: Compiled from ABCL, BCCRB, and BCFA national directories, reports, ephemera, and other sources.

will be clinics in Washington, Cleveland, Detroit, St. Paul, Minneapolis, Milwaukee, Denver, St. Louis, Los Angeles, San Francisco, San Diego, Portland, Seattle, Spokane and Butte," she had made no concrete plans for expansion. Though she also claimed in New York newspapers that her Washington confederates were ready to open "the minute I say the word," the floodgates did not open, possibly because Sanger's clinic was quickly raided. She and her staff were arrested, tried, and sentenced to short prison terms. No clinic opened in Washington, D.C., or any of those cities, save St. Paul, Minnesota. There, founder Sylvie Thygeson recalled that it "wasn't designated a birth control clinic. It was just an office, a room where we met and had lectures. We lectured on the desirability of birth control, tried to educate people to the idea of having too many people in the world." Extremely informal, it was also clandestine, as Thygeson explained, "Because it was so strictly against the law, we weren't printing it nor advertising it nor doing anything public about it. You don't do something that is against the ordinances of your city and the laws of your state. You don't do something like that in the open."[5] No records of this clinic survive, and it is unclear whether the St. Paul activists provided contraceptives.

When she opened the BCCRB, seven years after Brownsville, Sanger consciously created a model clinic, a viable organization that abided by the law. It was furnished with care, resembling a doctor's office with homey touches. The bureau employed a doctor, under whose license the clinic operated, as well as clerical workers and nurses. The bureau was a one-stop shop—it offered medical examinations, prescriptions, diaphragms, and contraceptive jelly on the premises. It also kept detailed statistics on patient progress. On her national speaking tours in the 1920s, Sanger exhorted women's clubs and medical men to join the birth control movement, organize leagues, and create clinics modeled on the BCCRB's mix of professionalism and female concern. The bureau model fit Sanger's philosophy that every woman should have the right to birth control knowledge, that the more economically fortunate women should help the poor secure that knowledge, and that the actual treatment of patients should be undertaken by physicians.[6]

In the 1920s, Sanger, the ABCL, and other activists formed independent clinics in major cities like New York, Chicago, Los Angeles, Baltimore, Detroit, San Francisco, Denver, Miami, and Philadelphia. While each was somewhat unique, they had much in common. The Indianapolis Maternal Health Clinic, though founded in 1934, offers an example of a typical independent clinic. The Indianapolis Maternal Health League was founded in 1932 with help from an ABCL organizer who worked to drum up interest and create a viable organization. In December of 1933 they organized a clinic, located in the Meridan Life Building in downtown Indianapolis, staffed by a paid physician (male) and nurses (female). Open only a few hours per week at first, the clinic restricted admission to married women who had been referred by a physician or social agency. They also would see only women who had borne at least two children, unless they had a serious medical condition. Patients who could pay were charged $1.25 for the service; those unable to pay were treated for free. To raise the operating costs of $1,800 to $2,400 per year, the league charged membership fees, patient fees, held fund-raising teas, and sent mail appeals.[7]

The Indianapolis clinic's main expenses were staff salaries and contraceptive supplies. The lay women who organized the clinic left medical policy to a small, male-dominated group of doctors while they assumed fiscal and administrative responsibility. The Indianapolis Maternal Health League also operated a medical referral service for women who lived outside the city, as well as a speakers bureau. Treating approximately five hundred new patients a year, Indianapolis's clientele was largely white (75–89 percent), with a smaller percentage of African American patients (11–25 percent). Most patients came to the clinic for economic reasons (75 percent); the rest came because of eugenic, social, or health concerns. In 1936 the league expanded its work to include statewide organizing. Renamed the Indiana Maternal Health League, it worked to foster leagues in other Indiana cities and developed a working relationship with the national activists.[8]

Without the backing of a respected institution, independent clinics often attracted criticism. Many who opposed birth control charged that clinics provided abortions, or that they encouraged promiscuity by treating unmarried women. Clinic founders used their reputations to deflect such criticism, but the risk was ever present that instead of bringing prestige to a controversial movement, the controversy would tarnish the founder's social standing. To hedge their bets, many independent clinics allied themselves with leading medical men and worked cooperatively rather than competitively with doctors.

Without advertising, independent clinics would not attract many patients. They relied upon word of mouth, collaborating with social service agencies, public health nurses, and others who worked with the poor to secure referrals. Some clinics used traditional publicity methods, taking out advertisements, printing business cards with hours and locations, holding public meetings on contraception and women's health, or meeting with neighborhood and church groups to encourage attendance. Press coverage brought in patients, so many leagues issued releases to trumpet clinic openings, annual meetings, and fund-raising drives. Others lobbied reporters to encourage colorful articles to promote the clinic. While some activists feared that press exposure would awaken opposition, they generally made no effort to keep the clinic's existence secret.

Birth control activists were free to shape the independent clinic as they pleased. Many establishments were decorated in homey styles, with pictures of babies on the walls, flowers, cribs, and toys to accommodate patients with children. They created lending libraries of birth control and sex education books for their patients and some operated car services to bring patients to and from their appointments.[9] Independent clinics bent their efforts to making it easy for patients to find and use the facility. Clinics ranged in professionalism, from a one-room cottage in Houston, furnished with an old kitchen table and a privacy curtain, to St. Louis's clinic, which had "aspects of a miniature hospital."[10] While the clinics tried to maintain a medical setting to instill confidence in their patients, they wanted patients to feel both safe and comfortable.

The independent clinic was the most common model in the 1920s and 1930s. Drawing on the charity experience of its women activists and the cooperation of paid or volunteer physicians, these clinics required a commitment of time and funds from their founders. Independent clinics were easier to create in urban areas, where both activists and patients were more numerous. They were rarely established in smaller cities. While the birth control leagues behind the clinics might have only a handful of members, finding a sufficient number of activists to foster clinics throughout even a single state was difficult, and the chances of populating an entire country with independent clinics would have required massive organization and fund-raising. Independent clinics were at their best when they introduced birth control to an area where it had not been known before; activists were needed to prove its worth, to lobby the local medical and political leaders, to raise funds to operate it, and to build public demand. Expanding this kind of service to cover an entire nation was inefficient and all but impossible to organize on limited funds.

Institutional Clinics

The most common institutional hosts for birth control clinics were hospitals, settlement houses, and public health agencies.[11] One could argue that each of these institutions offered the best home for birth control, as each was invested in improving the health and lives of working-class women. None of these organizations, however, saw birth control as their primary mission, or even as a very important secondary aim. Activists had to work hard to convince doctors, administrators, and officials that offering birth control was worth trying. Most of the time activists had to raise funds to entice the institutions to participate, but the results were not always worth the expense.

Early efforts to found institutional clinics in the 1920s focused on hospitals and settlement houses. Activists hoped that hospitals would offer birth control as an outpatient dispensary service alongside other services designed to serve the poor. Physicians who supported birth control saw hospital-based clinics as a means to assure medical control over contraception and to thwart efforts by lay women to dabble in medicine. Locating clinics in settlements grew out of alliances between social workers and society women. What made settlements different from other women's groups that founded clinics was that they did not form independent birth control leagues in order to found a clinic. Instead they used the mantle of the settlement. Despite a lot of activity in the 1920s, neither hospitals nor settlements proved interested enough in birth control to replace independent clinics.

In the late 1930s, birth control activists sought to take advantage of the maternal and infant welfare funding authorized by the 1935 Social Security Act to foster public health clinics at the state level. The economic rationales used for birth control were not new, but the Depression fostered the new notion that the government bore some responsibility to ameliorate poverty. Birth control activists argued that the best curb for rising relief spending was a combination of financial assistance and contraceptives. Birth control advocates argued that because the public funded relief programs, it had an interest in keeping the family size of those on relief manageable. A Pennsylvania Birth Control Federation flyer bluntly asked: "Mr. & Mrs. Taxpayer—How many children would you add to your family if you were absolutely dependent on public relief?" It went on to estimate that 280,000 people on relief in 1933 bore 4,840 babies at a cost to the government that year alone of almost $400,000. "Think what the cumulative cost to Philadelphia will be—for maintenance—for education—for hospitalization—of these children in the years to come."[12]

Whether founded in hospitals or settlement houses in the 1920s, or in city health departments in the 1930s, institutional clinics had some commonalities. They were usually organized by activists who formed a committee or subcommittee of the main organization. These activists may have been men and women just as committed to birth control as those who founded independent clinics, but the difference was that they had less control. Their plans had to be ratified by the officers, board, or membership of an entire organization, which often meant overcoming opposition from Catholic members, doctors hostile to birth control, or those who believed that other issues were more important.

Because they had less autonomy, many institutional clinics were content to serve a small clientele, culled from those already served by the institution. Hospitals would only accept existing patients in their birth control service; public health clinics might only accept women who had been screened by a visiting nurse, and settlements might limit access to neighborhood women who already participated in their programs. Publicity was often a sore spot with such institutions. They did not want to attract large numbers of outsiders clamoring for the services, nor did they want adverse publicity to threaten their mission or endanger donor relations. Hence, many institutions, particularly hospitals, demanded that the birth control movement keep their clinics a secret, seeking "no publicity." Others abruptly terminated services if opposition surfaced.[13]

Institutional clinics rejected close ties with birth control activists, seeking to maintain a "safe" distance from controversy. If questioned, some denied publicly that they had a birth control clinic, convincing themselves that what they did was not akin to an independent clinic. Chase Dispensary superintendent Dr. B. Henry Mason defended his service after it was raided by Waterbury, Connecticut, police in 1937: "It was not a birth control clinic in the accepted sense," Mason argued, "where any woman who doesn't want children may go." He saw his service as medical, while he characterized independent clinics as lax and unprofessional.[14] Many doctors were particularly suspicious of Margaret Sanger and the ABCL, hastening to assure the public that their work was not linked—even when it was. Dr. Robert Latou Dickinson, founder of a number of hospital-based clinics in New York City in the 1920s, publicly criticized Sanger's BCCRB as a propaganda tool. Privately he needed Sanger's help to get enough diaphragms for his patients, and when his clinics were sparsely attended, he courted her to obtain clinical data for his work. Dr. George M. Cooper, director of North Carolina's Department of Health, accepted funds from birth control activist Dr. Clarence Gamble to open "prevenceptive" clinics at health departments in 1937, but became incensed when a reporter linked his work to the BCCRB (Clarence Gamble sat on its advisory board). Cooper denied any contact with Sanger, writing her directly that any link with her organization would jeopardize his entire program.[15]

Institutional clinics had good reason to be cautious, especially when they received public funds. Opposition to birth control clinics, usually from Catholics, was a constant threat, as were complaints about the immoral use of tax dollars, the suspicion that clinics offered abortion, and the assumption that providing birth control was illegal. While they may have believed in the efficacy of birth control, most institutional clinics lacked the top-down commitment of a league created specifically to promote the cause. Institutional clinic boards were often more concerned with appeasing critics than providing services. When trouble came to these clinics, they were far more vulnerable than independent clinics. When one hospital clinic was attacked by the local Catholic bishop because it was located at a publicly funded hospital in Cincinnati, rather than fight, the hospital board encouraged Dr. Elizabeth Campbell to move the clinic to a private hospital.[16] In cities with large Catholic populations, activists did not even try to secure interest from city or state governments for a publicly supported clinic. It was in the South, where few Catholics lived, that public health officers first agreed to offer birth control, in some cases hoping to use it to reduce the mortality and the birth rates of poor whites and African Americans.[17]

Hospitals

Placing birth control in hospitals seemed a logical fit, given their growing importance in American health care delivery. By the 1920s, privately owned hospitals, run either by nonprofit charities and corporations or as for-profit businesses, were consumer-based entities that attracted patients with promises of modern services and equipment. Hospital-based obstetrical care was one of the fastest growing services. Hospitals were attractive to birth control activists because they were already nationally distributed to reach both urban and rural patients.[18] To convince socially conservative doctors, activists downplayed feminist and radical arguments for birth control, instead pressing claims that birth control would improve women's health and reduce infant and maternal mortality rates. This was a difficult challenge, for several factors worked against them.

Hospitals had become specialists in dramatic cures, surgery, and interventionist obstetrical care, while de-emphasizing preventive medicine. Doctors preferred to leave the social and economic conditions that brought on diseases—conditions such as unemployment, poor housing, overcrowding, or poor sanitation—to social workers to solve. Doctors wanted to be responsible only for the medical treatment of diseases, leaving public health experts to contain and prevent them. They were interested in reducing infant and maternal mortality, but they focused on licensing, and then limiting, the role of nonphysician birth attendants like midwives.[19] The activists' argument that birth control could improve maternal health was viewed neither by doctors as a medical issue nor by social workers as an educational one, and thus it got the full attention of neither group.

Of more concern was that by the 1920s, hospital services were stratified by class and were highly competitive. Likening private hospitals to ocean liners, with first-class and steerage accommodations, historian Rosemary Stevens argued that the "first-class" sections of hospitals were expanding, if often only half-filled, while the crowded wards for the poor were decreasing in size despite increased demand. Hospital administrators saw little profit in expanding services for those who could not pay. Even when working-class patients managed to get a bed in a hospital, the wards were "dirty, crowded, in ill repair, short of essential supplies . . . understaffed, and lacking in standard equipment."[20] With birth control patients drawn from the same unwelcome population of charity cases, activists had trouble convincing hospitals to expend resources in this direction.

The first person to tackle the introduction of birth control clinics in hospitals was Dr. Robert Latou Dickinson, who worked in New York City to establish hospital clinics in response to the challenge posed by Sanger's BCCRB. In order to wrest birth control from the meddling of lay women, Dickinson's Committee on Maternal Health (CMH) offered contraceptive services in twelve New York City hospitals between 1923 and 1932. Participating hospitals agreed to prescribe contraceptives to existing and needy patients, to gather statistics on the patients and on the effectiveness of methods, and to report the data to the committee. Situated within the hospitals' existing outpatient departments, these clinics saw poor and charity patients. Hospital staff, wary of "charity abuse," used moral rulers to decide which patients to accept, seeking to treat only the "honest" and "deserving" poor. They refused to allow any publicity through the ABCL, for fear that the hospital "might take umbrage or alarm . . . if their names appeared in the press."[21]

Handicapped from the start, Dickinson's attempt failed, foundering on the reluctance of hospitals to welcome the service and on the unwillingness of patients to submit to the process. Birth control was not yet widely accepted in the medical profession, and in their zeal to protect themselves legally, the committee's clinics adopted an admission policy so rigid that it discouraged participation. In at least one case, Mount Sinai superintendent Robert Frank reported that while physicians were willing to refer women for therapeutic abortions, they would not refer them to the contraceptive clinic for fear of being second guessed by the admission committee.[22] As one patient described the process, "You have to be a terrible invalid . . . and then three doctors must agree that it is necessary."[23] Some doctors who worked in the hospitals that hosted clinics preferred to refer their patients to the BCCRB, where referrals were quietly and eagerly accepted. The CMH also interpreted New York State law very strictly, hamstringing its efforts. It simply could not gather enough data to make valid conclusions. After three years of work, the nine clinics under the committee's coordination had submitted only 124 patient histories to Dickinson. Many were incomplete and useless for research. Dickinson characterized the patients as "shy of such places and the doctors mostly timorous." By contrast the BCCRB, located in the same city, had gathered nine hundred patient records in its first year. Concerned by its inability to secure data, the CMH did not loosen admission policies, but instead eventually gave up. Though the hospital clinics founded by the CMH limped along for years, they never became integral either to their institutions or to the birth control movement.[24]

The New York hospital clinics of the 1920s failed to offer a viable alternate to the independent clinic, but efforts continued to create the kind of hospital service that Dickinson envisioned. In 1929 a Cincinnati Committee on Maternal Health, modeled on Dickinson's original, opened a birth control clinic in the General Hospital's Obstetrical Department. Overseen by Dr. Elizabeth Campbell, the clinic admitted patients who had referrals from a doctor, minister, or social welfare agency, and saw approximately one thousand patients in its first two years. Operated by medical and lay staff, initial funding came from philanthropist and birth control activist Clarence J. Gamble. The lay committee handled fund-raising, attracted patients, and conducted follow-up work. As other hospital clinics would do, the Cincinnati Maternal Health Committee remained aloof from the birth control movement. It did not affiliate with the ABCL, Sanger's BCCRB, or the National Committee on Federal Legislation for Birth Control (NCFLBC), though it did affiliate with the CMH. Despite efforts to operate quietly, it was attacked by Cincinnati's Catholic archbishop John T. McNicholas in 1931. The bishop questioned the propriety of using a publicly funded hospital for an "immoral" purpose. Rather than defend its rights to exist at public expense, the committee voluntarily moved to the privately funded Children's Hospital.[25]

Cincinnati's reliance on lay participation in an institutional clinic was repeated in other cities throughout the 1930s. Hospitals would provide staff and facilities if they could get financial backing from outside activists. For birth control activists, this partnership offered the security of a respected institution and guaranteed good relations with local doctors. For the hospital it offered a minimal commitment to a charity program that many did not value. Hard hit by the Depression, contributions to hospitals were down, and paying patients were far outnumbered by requests for charity care.[26] Because adding more charity services was unattractive to administrators, birth control could only get into hospitals if outside activists pushed it in. Activists would secure allies among the hospital's medical staff, then offer its board a plan that expected very little from the hospital. The hospital provided space and staffing, and the lay activists managed funding, supplies, record keeping, and administration. In Waterbury, the link between the hospital and the clinic was so tenuous that lay volunteers took patient records home each night rather than keep them on the hospital premises.[27]

In theory, hospital clinics offered their patients a wider range of services than independent birth control clinics. When birth control was offered as part of a larger woman's health program, patients could receive treatment for all their ailments, whether gynecological or not, at one time and place. At independent clinics, patients might be given a physical and gynecological examination. If disorders were found, they were referred to another clinic for treatment. At the Woman's Hospital clinic in Detroit, patients were found suffering from conditions ranging from tumors, relaxed perineums, lacerated cervixes, retroversions, prolapsed uterus, endocervitis, cystocele, and rectocele. Other clinics detected cervical or uterine cancer during medical examinations, and while none reported figures as high as the Recreation Rooms Settlement clinic in New York, where 47.6 percent of patients had some form of pelvic pathology, the BCFA reported that 6 percent of patients nationwide had medical conditions that required a referral for immediate treatment.[28]

Hospital clinics could have served as "one-stop" treatment centers for working-class women, but there was no financial incentive to offer such services to patients unable to pay for them. To keep down costs hospitals used complex admission policies to discourage all but the truly desperate from using their services. An example of the kinds of red tape that dogged hospital-based clinics can be found at the Sloan Hospital in New York City, one of the CMH affiliates. Patients could not simply walk up to the clinic and request advice. Instead, they had to be selected by a member of the hospital's social service department using strict medical criteria to screen their cases. Once selected, the patient was evaluated by a staff doctor. If he—and most hospital doctors were men—approved, the patient was then referred to Dr. Jean Corwin, who again screened the patient for medical need. If the social service department, the staff doctor, and Dr. Corwin all agreed, then the patient was sent to Dr. E. Everett Bunzel, who performed another examination and prescribed a contraceptive. A similar policy was in place at Mount Sinai Hospital in New York, where OB/GYN chief Dr. Max D. Meyer treated patients only after they were cleared for economic need and were referred by another Mount Sinai physician.[29] It is not surprising that most patients, rather than face such a gauntlet, sought the more relaxed atmosphere of the independent clinic, where they could be interviewed, evaluated, and treated in one visit.

While many hospital clinics worked in conjunction with the local birth control activists, few had strong connections with state or national birth control leagues. In some cases, especially in the 1920s, hospitals set up their own informal referral services without telling any birth control activists. This could lead to embarrassing meetings, such as in 1932, when BCCRB field worker Clara Louise McGraw tried to persuade St. Luke's Hospital in St. Louis to host a clinic in conjunction with the Missouri Maternal Health Association. The chaplain and superintendent of the hospital informed her, "We have been running a birth control clinic at St. Luke's Hospital for the past two years or more. It has been done in a quiet but constructive manner."[30] Clinics so quiet that local and national activists did not know they existed could not have been well-attended. Typical of the tenuous relationship between hospitals and birth control activists was the situation at Atlanta's Henry W. Grady Memorial Hospital's Gynecology Department. The hospital had sporadically offered birth control services to both African Americans and whites from 1930 to 1939, through a prenatal clinic funded by the Jewish Social Service League. Though Dr. Ingram, the clinic director, wanted to expand the clinic's work, he was unwilling to work with local birth control activists, opposed any lay control or involvement with his clinic, and refused efforts to publicize the clinic through the national birth control movement.[31] Most hospitals agreed that keeping a "low profile" was in their best interests. In French Camp, California, the San Joaquin Hospital opened the Stockton Mother's Health Clinic in a Catholic-dominated neighborhood in 1934. Prodded several times by the BCCRB to list the clinic in a national directory, the hospital refused, fearing that it would bring negative attention to their work. When the hospital finally relented in 1936, they buried all mention of the hospital itself, listing the clinic simply under the name of its medical director. They continued to refuse any formal affiliation with the BCCRB, promising only vaguely to "consider" affiliating at some point in the distant future.[32] "No publicity" followed the names of many of the hospital clinics in the national directories, meaning that while the BCCRB and ABCL knew the clinic existed, they were not to make it generally known. These clinics did not want walk-in patients, shunned any association with the birth control movement, and wanted to provide birth control on their own terms.

The lack of commitment to birth control at hospitals is demonstrated well by the Pasadena Woman's Hospital clinic, for which we have a richer documentary record than most. A small nonprofit maternity hospital, the Woman's Hospital was founded by a group of wealthy lay women to serve the underprivileged in Pasadena. In 1931, the board was approached by an agent of Dr. Clarence J. Gamble (who unsuccessfully tried to remain anonymous), who offered to cover the costs of a birth control clinic. Gamble wanted to provide the hospital with seed money to establish the clinic, expecting that it would eventually become self-supporting. He proposed a model in which the hospital board advertised the clinic, secured volunteer workers, kept records, and brought in donations and patient fees to eventually cover its costs. The board agreed to Gamble's terms and for three years the clinic limped along with little internal support and practically no funding other than that provided by Gamble. When Gamble criticized the low patient counts and bombarded the board with a continuing stream of ideas on attracting more patients and publicity, he ran up against a wall of apathy. His agents found hospital board members interested only in securing more of Gamble's money. They were unwilling to seek funds for the clinic from anywhere else for fear that publicity might damage the hospital's general fund-raising efforts. Gamble's tactics, including pushes for advertisements and aggressive work among Pasadena social work agencies, clashed with the hospital board's aims. They saw the clinic as a small, relatively unimportant part of their larger work. Much less committed to birth control than Gamble or his staff, the hospital board refused to prioritize its birth control service. When Gamble threatened to pull his funding if they did not agree to take a greater role, board director Florence Banning refused, claiming that she would do nothing to jeopardize potential donations. Banning believed that birth control activists should raise funds for the clinic and donate them to the hospital. She was equally uninterested in Gamble's suggestion that they press patients to pay a portion of the treatment costs, arguing that their patients were too poor to do so. Banning thought that forcing women to pay for birth control (as opposed to their maternity bills), would be counterproductive and instead entreated him to continue fully funding the clinic. Faced with this intransigence, Gamble ceased his support, advising them to create a lay birth control league in Pasadena to fund the clinic. Eventually a local group was formed to raise funds for several area clinics, including the Pasadena Woman's Hospital, and the clinics were continued into the 1940s.[33]

Despite the efforts of activists like Dickinson, Gamble, and others and growing acceptance that birth control was a useful tool of preventive medicine, it became clear to most birth control activists that hospital clinics would never replace independent clinics. Hospitals were unwilling to assume fiscal responsibility for ensuring access to contraception for those who could not afford it. They were not interested in charity work, especially if it was controversial, and felt that offering such services opened them to ridicule or to charges of immorality. In an era when most hospital and medical associations fought against "socialized" programs that promised to offer health coverage to all Americans, and with no financial incentive to expand its services for birth control, hospitals had little interest in providing birth control at their own expense. They preferred that the government or charity sector take responsibility for the health of the indigent.

Settlement Houses

If hospitals were uninterested in giving medical services to the poor, one might expect that institutions dedicated to helping the working class would be. Despite the affinity between birth control and settlement activists, only thirty-seven birth control clinics were founded in settlement houses between 1916 and 1939, between 5 to 15 percent of the total clinics in any given year. Most were located in a handful of industrial cities in the Northeast and Midwest.

The appeal of the settlement house as a host for a birth control clinic was understandable. As Charlotte Delafield Marsh of the New York City Committee of the ABCL wrote, "We concluded that the most practical work on hand was to open as many birth control centers as possible near the homes of poor mothers and that settlement houses were the logical places."[34] Settlements, established in the immigrant neighborhoods, were already working with the communities that activists wanted to reach. They had relationships with the leaders and a track record of providing both education and health care. Financed and operated by the same cadre of society women who supported birth control, the social networks of the sponsors overlapped. Some of the nation's earliest birth control clinics, particularly in Chicago, were located in settlements. The Illinois Birth Control League (IBCL) was initially created in 1923 as a committee of the Chicago Woman's Club, and was led by lay women and prominent women physicians who resided at Hull House. They saw birth control as a way to address the educative and health problems facing their clients. Clinics were formed in several nearby settlements and the IBCL also opened an independent clinic, catering to wealthier patients. Funds raised there were used to offset costs at the settlement clinics. Dr. Rachelle Yarros and a handful of women doctors volunteered their services, keeping overhead low. The settlements provided the premises and funds to purchase contraceptives, and worked with charitable organizations in Chicago to raise the rest of the money.[35]

The social service groups that adopted the IBCL clinics did more than just write a check. The Chicago Woman's Aid Society undertook financial responsibility for the lay staff of the Jewish People's Institute clinic, which treated several thousand patients annually. The IBCL provided volunteer doctors and set medical policy and standards. Because of their volunteers, by 1937 the clinic had made a profit of almost one thousand dollars, which the society donated to the IBCL. When that clinic became overcrowded, it was the society, not the IBCL, that developed plans to open another clinic nearby, working with local Jewish charities to sponsor the House of Social Service clinic in 1939.[36]

By the 1930s, New York was another locus of settlement-sponsored clinics, as the ABCL's New York City Committee found thirteen willing settlements to house their clinics. Building close ties with social work organizations, the New York Committee hired four nurses and a part-time social worker, who were shared between the clinics. They paid physicians a token salary and covered the costs of contraceptive supplies. In New York, the settlement contributed only space and the services of a nurse. The thirteen New York settlement clinics had seen twelve thousand patients by 1935 and eighteen thousand by 1937, an impressive figure, given that the BCCRB also operated in New York.[37]

The examples of Chicago and New York show that successful collaborations between birth control, settlement, and social service activists could result in vibrant and popular clinics, operated at low cost. But the eighteen New York and Chicago clinics make up almost half of the total number of settlement clinics founded.[38] The others were scattered in settlements across the country and were not unified by a single coordinating birth control league. Most saw very few patients. The problem for settlement clinics, and the reason that they never became an important institutional sponsor for clinics, may have been more one of timing than a structural problem with the model.

The settlement movement was dying in the 1920s and 1930s. As the infusion of new immigrants diminished and was then cut off by restrictive laws, the popular Americanization programs offered by settlements seemed less relevant. And with the great migration of African Americans from the South into the settlement's neighborhoods, activists wrestled with the challenge of providing an interracial and interclass community center. Few succeeded. Some settlements moved out when African Americans began to dominate the neighborhood, while others found that when they welcomed African Americans their white clients began to disappear, creating de facto segregation. In addition, by the mid to late 1930s, the dramatic increase in New Deal social services made settlement house programs seem old-fashioned and unappealing to volunteers, and the movement rapidly declined.[39]

Funding was another factor that affected a settlement's willingness to work with birth control activists. While initially supported through private donations, by the 1930s settlements and other community organizations began to get the bulk of their funds through community-based fund-raising organizations like the Community Chest. While this relieved settlement boards of the worry of raising operating budgets, it impacted the services they offered. Community Chest officials had the power to veto individual programs when reviewing the overall budget for a settlement and rather than face tough scrutiny, many simply dropped anything controversial from their budgets. Even in instances where they already offered birth control, settlements were unlikely to include it in their budget requests. New York Committee head Charlotte Delafield Marsh hoped settlements would "eventually take over the responsibility for financing the centers. . . . We will then be able to use our own funds to start new centers, which will in turn become self-supporting—thus enabling us to enter new fields."[40] While Marsh and the committee doubled the number of settlement-based clinics between 1931 and 1939, none of the hosts took the next step of taking over fiscal responsibility for the work, limiting the ability of the activists to expand clinical service.

Like hospital clinics, settlement clinics drew patients from a limited pool. Most were small operations, centered around a specific neighborhood. Women were unlikely to travel far to attend these clinics, which were advertised mostly to social workers. Settlement clinic patients were the same women who used the settlement's other services. Birth control activists who founded clinics essentially won access to court the settlement's members; they could not advertise the clinics citywide.[41]

The decline of settlements and their neighborhood focus limited their usefulness as a means to spread birth control to all American women. Where the settlement clinics were active, such as in New York and Chicago, they provided something that neither hospital nor independent clinics did—an integration of social, educational, and medical services geared toward helping the poor without stigmatizing them. But like other institutional clinics, settlements were not primarily birth control organizations, and most were unwilling to run risks to provide these services to their clients.

Government-Sponsored Clinics

Despite activists' dreams of government-supplied birth control, in the 1920s and 1930s the federal government refused to accept responsibility for health care. This failure will be detailed in chapter 6. Rebuffed at the federal level, birth control activists turned to state and city health departments and relief boards. There they found only limited success. Only a handful of government agencies provided birth control in the 1920s and early 1930s: the Los Angeles County Health Department and the Michigan Emergency Relief Administration were the most prominent. In the late 1930s, birth control activists found success lobbying state boards of health in South Carolina, North Carolina, Virginia, and West Virginia. But there the drive foundered, stalled by opposition from the medical profession and an unwillingness to fund a service that some found morally objectionable.

Of the publicly funded birth control clinics, none stands out more as a model of how contraceptives could have been integrated into public health services than the Los Angeles County Health Department's program. Very little has been written about this effort, which was headed by Dr. John Larrabee Pomeroy. Under Pomeroy, Los Angeles's Health Department was noted for its aggressive administration over a system of decentralized health centers and for the outstanding results it achieved in lowering both infant mortality and the death rate. With a background in tuberculosis treatment at both public and private sanatoriums, Pomeroy took charge in 1915, opening twelve regional health centers that offered emergency surgery, a range of specialty services (including dental, venereal disease, and tuberculosis clinics), treatment for noncontagious diseases, and pre- and postnatal instruction. After 1927, these clinics provided contraceptive advice as well. Many of the services offered by the Health Department went beyond its legal mandate, but Pomeroy allied with private physicians, convincing them to volunteer their time at the health centers. Before 1932, patients were charged nominal fees (between ten and fifty cents), which were pooled and used by the doctors for charitable purposes.[42]

Pomeroy's results, measured by the reduction of death rates, were impressive. The infant mortality rate in 1915 was at 96 per one thousand births. Within that, pockets of extremely high mortality lurked. Infants of Mexican descent died at a rate of 500 per one thousand births. As health centers were installed throughout the county, the infant mortality rate fell to 30 per one thousand births, lower than the national average of 43. Though Mexican Americans still died more frequently than white and Japanese American infants did, the improvement was remarkable. Lower rates of adult deaths from contagious diseases were also reported.[43]

Dr. Nadina Reinstein Kavinoky served as the liaison between the county health department and Los Angeles birth control activists. Kavinoky, a Swiss-born gynecologist, headed both the health centers and the less formal Mother's Conferences (meetings between doctors and patients at regularly scheduled times), where birth control was provided. She represented the Health Department at conferences organized by the ABCL and BCCRB, reported on the county's clinics to national activists, and likely treated the majority of patients at the clinics. Of thirty-three clinics in Los Angeles County, Kavinoky was either the medical director or a staff physician at eighteen of them. In addition to her work for the county, she also served at the White Memorial Hospital clinic, the Pasadena Woman's Hospital clinic, and the Pasadena General Hospital clinic. Kavinoky spoke to civic and women's groups on birth control, supported the repeal of the Comstock

Act, taught contraceptive technique to medical students at the College of Medical Evangelists, and reported on the California clinics at international birth control conferences and meetings of the American Public Health Association.[44]

While the procedures at the county's service were similar to what occurred at independent or hospital clinics, there were differences. At independent clinics, the process was usually patient-driven; that is, a patient appealed to the clinic for information. In the Los Angeles County public health clinics, county nurses, social workers, and doctors identified birth control prospects as they came across them in their regular work. Kavinoky claimed that 70 percent of her fifteen hundred patients had "high motivation" and she expected a good success rate from them. Of the remaining 30 percent, she admitted, "the initiative is not with the patient . . . it is frequently with the physician in the tuberculosis or venereal disease divisions" who referred them.[45] The Los Angeles County clinics did not force contraception on any patient. While the county nurses would visit a patient who did not report for a scheduled follow-up, nurses were instructed to close the case if the patient objected to contraception because of religious convictions or if she had lost interest.

Patients at the Los Angeles County clinics had to present both economic and medical indications for contraception in order to be treated. For admission to any county-sponsored medical service, a patient also had to pass a residency test. Once inside, the procedure of examinations, diaphragm fitting, and patient training was very much the same as at an independent clinic. Where the county excelled was in the numbers of clinics they were able to scatter around the region, enabling poor women to get advice in their own neighborhoods. Potential patients were screened into birth control services when they attended tuberculosis clinics, venereal disease clinics, and infant welfare programs, and the integration between the services seems to have resulted in higher patient numbers than other government-funded clinics attained. In the first three years of the program, some five hundred patients were seen each year, with a success rate of 96 percent.[46]

Los Angeles County's experience in the 1930s also illustrates the risks of publicly funded clinics. The pleasant relations that Pomeroy had with the medical profession from 1915 to 1931 were uncommon, if not unique. In most cities public health work was controversial, as the medical profession fiercely opposed any encroachments on their livelihood. With the onset of the Depression, Los Angeles County's unique experiment in cooperative health care broke down. In November 1933, Kavinoky informed Sanger that "we came very close to losing all the Mothers' Clinics in the Los Angeles County Health Department," due to the inevitable budget cuts, but also because of "pressure and fear of preventive health work on the part of our private practitioners."[47] There had always been some opposition from the medical community to the County Health Department's work, but with hard economic times it crystallized. The doctors who had volunteered at the "curative" clinics revolted. As their practices declined with their patients' income, physicians balked at being asked to give free treatments at the county clinics to the same people who used to pay them in their offices. Claiming that the county social workers accepted anyone, even "millionaires" for free services, the physicians sought to dismantle the public health center system. They withdrew their support for the extra clinics that the Health Department instituted and forced the department to drop any extracurricular patients or services. This meant that health centers could now only admit people with communicable diseases who were eligible for county aid. They next closed most of the county health centers entirely through "the San Fernando Plan," which privatized public health by using government funds to pay physicians to treat indigent patients in their own offices rather than support freestanding health centers. Opponents of this plan predicted that once the economy improved, the same physicians who now clamored for county patients would refuse to treat the indigent at the low fees paid by the government. But by then, the public health system would be decimated.[48] Without legislative authority and medical support, Pomeroy could not operate the expanded service. Once it became financially onerous, physicians withdrew their support.

Contraceptive services at the health centers were not spared this attack, though surprisingly, physicians who opposed the clinics did not do so for moral or religious reasons—again, it was money that roused their ire. A group of physicians from Huntington Park, angered by their declining incomes, sought to reduce the city's contribution to the health centers and targeted several programs for elimination. They specifically condemned the contraceptive clinic on the grounds that it took away from their private practice. Pomeroy defended the service by arguing that its chief purpose was the reduction of tuberculosis and syphilis, but that it also helped to reduce abortions and related maternal deaths. He also argued that the seventy-four patients at the Huntington Park Health Center that year had all met the economic criteria for treatment and could not have afforded private care.

Though Pomeroy succeeded in convincing Huntington Park to continue its funding, similar criticisms from the Los Angeles County Medical Society and from the newly created Public Health Physicians' League made it impossible for the health centers to continue as before. After the San Fernando Plan was implemented in 1932, the county's contraceptive clinics, just as all of their services, were limited to indigent women suffering from either tuberculosis or venereal disease. To secure birth control for the many patients newly denied care, Kavinoky sought her own public-private partnership, forging agreements with individual physicians to take indigent contraceptive patients in their private offices for a fee (usually between two and three dollars). She then organized committees of lay women to raise the funds needed to cover these fees. Though by 1937 Kavinoky proclaimed herself satisfied with these results, the majority of patients in Los Angeles County were no longer being treated in a clinical setting.[49]

In its first seven years, Los Angeles County had the kind of program that birth control activists wanted to see in place across the nation. It offered birth control as part of a large-scale maternal and infant welfare program without any serious controversy, even in an area with a large Catholic population. But the program was on shaky ground, going far beyond the Health Department's legal mandate. Once the medical profession turned against the public health centers, the Los Angeles experiment was dismantled.[50] No other public health program operated on the scale that Los Angeles County did, though most were equally fragile. Because they were located in city health departments or sponsored by county relief agencies, in many cases it is difficult to determine how much support the government agency actually provided the clinics. In 1937, the ABCL identified two levels of government support, reporting eighty-five clinics funded by various government entities and forty-three that were privately funded, but worked out of government offices. As was often the case when dealing with government clinics, the ABCL did not reveal the location of the clinics; it just claimed that five unnamed states had "fairly well developed programs."[51]

The level of support that clinics received from a municipal, county, or state government varied. In some places, the clinics received full funding and integration into regular services, as was the case in Los Angeles. In other places, like Ponca City, Oklahoma, the mayor and health board provided space, salaries, and supplies, but established a lay organization to officially "run" the clinic. In Detroit, Josephine Gorman, a board member of the Birth Control League, used her position as secretary to Mayor Frank Murphy to convince him to allow social workers and visiting nurses to refer indigent patients to the league's Harper Hospital birth control clinic. In still other places, the government's only contribution was to allow a birth control league to use its space on off hours.[52]

In Michigan, a wide variety of government agencies offered birth control services, but what linked all these clinics together was the agitation of the Michigan Maternal Health League, the lay activist organization. Their lobbying was critical to pressuring the County Emergency Relief Administration to provide contraceptive service, while in other cities they convinced the Poor Commission, the Department of Public Welfare, or the Health Department to do so. Government support sometimes took the form of payments to independent clinics for treating relief patients.[53] While these services seem to have been increased in the late 1930s, many of them were ephemeral and crisis-driven, lasting only until economic conditions improved. Governments saw them as a stopgap measure to take pressure off families and to reduce the burden on their welfare rolls. When the economy began to improve, most were cut off without any notice. Of the seven government-funded programs in Michigan, only clinics in Cadillac and Ironwood were still in operation by 1939.[54]

The best example of a statewide program in the late 1930s is found in North Carolina, where an extensive campaign to include contraception in the public health program was begun in 1937. Funded not by Social Security grants to the Department of Health, but by birth control activist Clarence J. Gamble, the state authorized county health officers to add contraception to their existing services for the indigent. North Carolina used the grant money to pay Gamble's organizer to help county health units set up the service and cover the costs of supplies. That organizer, public health nurse Frances Roberta Pratt, traveled around the state visiting the county officers and setting up clinics, most of which were operated when the regular public health office was closed. These "prevenceptive" clinics served two purposes: to test an experimental contraceptive—foam powder—and to test the efficacy of statewide birth control delivery.[55]

In addition to the clinics, visiting nurses also offered contraceptive information to patients in their homes. Most clinic patients came via nurse referrals (67 percent), with the traditional sources of patients, social workers (12 percent), and private physicians (15 percent) responsible for smaller percentages. More than half of the patients treated (57 percent) obtained care at a county health center, but a significant minority (35 percent) received the care in their own homes. North Carolina's choice of contraceptives enabled them to split their program between home visitation and clinical settings because foam powder did not require a pelvic examination by a physician. Like Los Angeles, the North Carolina contraceptive program was driven by the public health staff, not the patients—contraception on demand was not offered.[56]

North Carolina was widely touted as the first test of a statewide program of publicly funded birth control, but it was not. The North Carolina clinics were not state funded. They were state-administered but funded through the private donation of a birth control activist with his own agenda. North Carolina spent no state funds on the program and many involved with it were uneasy about any public links with the birth control movement. They resisted the efforts of birth control activists to drum up attention to the program as a model for other public health departments. Like other institutional clinics, the North Carolina experiment saw few patients. Though 75 percent of the state's counties participated in the birth control experiment, creating fifty-six "prevenceptive" centers in only two years, only 1,311 patients were seen statewide, an average of under twelve patients per clinic per *year*. Likewise, the North Carolina clinics served multiple goals. For Gamble the focus was on testing the foam powder contraceptive. For the public health nurses and patients it was about preventing individual pregnancies. For the county health officers, it was a reduction in death rates and improvements to overall health. A few health officers adopted the program with the hope of reducing the population of poor blacks in their counties.[57]

The North Carolina clinics did not succeed by any measure. Because of Gamble's interest in testing foam powder contraceptives, clinics were encouraged (though not compelled) to use that method. While some prevenceptive centers rejected foam powder in favor of the more commonly used diaphragm/jelly combination, the majority used the unproven method and gathered data on its effectiveness.[58] Neither field workers nor patients were happy with foam powder, but they were pressured to continue using it in order to complete the clinical trials. One field worker threatened to quit in 1940, feeling that her orders to prescribe foam powder were jeopardizing the birth control program. After a rash of failures with foam powder, she requested, but was denied, the right to offer patients other contraceptive methods. Even as a contraceptive trial the program failed because individual health officers kept inadequate records. For a contraceptive clinic, the inability to prescribe the most effective contraceptive led to a high dropout rate, as patients became disillusioned. As an effort to convince the state to support the program, the North Carolina experiment was only moderately successful. When Gamble withdrew his funding in 1940, the state did not replace the funds; instead, each county health commissioner had to decide whether to use their own funds, close the clinic down, or raise private funds to keep it going. Many clinics were shut down, but some health commissioners managed to continue them. Some were funded by private individuals or women's organizations. Others charged patient fees. Though the number of patients treated at the remaining clinics eventually rose in the 1940s to about three thousand statewide, it never reached the potential number of patients that could have attended, given the statewide network of clinics.[59]

North Carolina's health officers did more than downplay their connection with the birth control movement; they actively denied it. When Roy Norton reported on the clinics at the 1938 meeting of the American Public Health Association, he claimed the impetus for the program "came as a result of hundreds of mothers, mostly of low economic status writing to the Board of Health asking for birth control information." He never mentioned Clarence Gamble, though as was his wont, Gamble had requested anonymity. After a mix-up linked the North Carolina clinics with Sanger's BCCRB, the press asked George Cooper, the state's director for the Division of Maternity and Infancy, about his relationship with Sanger. "She didn't have a dad-blamed thing to do with it, and we don't want any part of Margaret Sanger's advertising and controversy," he retorted.[60]

In South Carolina, a very different relationship was established between the birth control movement and the state. With a nation-leading maternal mortality rate of ninety-nine deaths per one thousand births, the State Medical Association formed a study group that concluded that at least 25 percent of those who died were "chronically unfit for the hazards of pregnancy." This led to a 1938 State Board of Health ruling enabling state doctors to prescribe contraceptives to at-risk women. South Carolina worked with the BCFA on much the same terms that North Carolina had worked with Gamble, but did so openly. The BCFA lent the state a public health nurse and provided the costs of the contraceptives used, but otherwise did not interfere in the state's administration of the health centers. As in North Carolina, each county health officer was offered the service and could choose whether or not to adopt it. In South Carolina the clinics were not separated from the regular public health centers, as in North Carolina. Director Robert Seibels reported: "We have no distinct 'birth control' clinics under public health nor do we plan to establish any. These patients receive this information when they need it and the prescription for their receiving it may be written by the physician conducting the tuberculosis clinic, a well-baby clinic or any activity of the county health office. Thus we have tried to integrate our pregnancy spacing advice into the public health program and have tried not to make it more important than any other of our activities or to neglect it when an indication arises."

South Carolina's contraceptive program, integrated into a larger effort of education and data gathering, proved effective in reducing maternal mortality, which declined by 30 percent to sixty-six deaths per one thousand births by 1940. But the state did not pay for it and, again, relatively few women used the service.[61]

National Models

Birth control clinics came in a variety of shapes, but the most practical was the independent clinic. Efforts to secure institutional support for contraceptives hinged on the willingness of the U.S. government to subsidize medical costs or on the charitable impulses of a hospital or settlement. As none of these institutional entities were as committed to birth control as its activists, few were willing to put in the long hours and work needed to fund the clinics, especially if they could shift responsibility elsewhere.

Judging both by their prevalence and by the numbers of patients treated, independent clinics were popular with both the activists who founded them and with the patients who used them. But they could not do it all. They were expensive, if not in dollars, then in time. Building a volunteer-based movement large enough to offer independent clinics to all women foundered against the sheer size and spread of the population. Independent clinics operated best in urban areas, where the population concentration provided both sufficient birth control activists *and* potential patients. In rural areas where the population was more sparsely settled and medical care difficult to obtain, there were neither enough activists nor physicians to staff small community clinics. Because travel beyond a few miles could be a great hardship for the rural poor, the independent clinic model could not succeed in distributing contraceptives to all the nation's women.

Birth control activists initially saw the independent clinic as an interim step; once they had demonstrated the utility of birth control as a health and welfare issue they believed the proper social and governmental agencies would take over. In practice, this was a much harder sell than they expected, as governments and hospitals were reluctant to take up the challenge, and those that did often did so grudgingly. In most cases where birth control leaders and philanthropists tried to include contraceptives into the existing programs of hospitals, settlement houses, and public health or emergency relief programs, they had to cover the costs of these programs. While birth control activists saw this as an investment that would result in an eventual takeover of the service by the institution, the institution saw it as evidence that they would not have to pay for these services. For most institutions, birth control was extracurricular; it was not a part of their general program and they would not let it compete with efforts to fund other programs. Birth control was still too controversial. It still attracted more negative attention than many institutional boards were willing to allow.

Institutional clinics were few and far between, and often temporary. Only independent birth control clinics accepted long-term and large-scale responsibility for running clinics, dealing with opposition, and funding the service. There was no widespread support for birth control clinics at the national level, neither from medical associations, hospital leagues, nor the federal government. Birth control's strongest support was local, whether in the form of an independent clinic, a city public health department, or a neighborhood settlement committed to serving its poor. Doctors, activists, and government officials were far more likely to recognize the need for birth control advice when it was presented in a tangible form, not in abstract argument. But without official backing, the effort to create an effective national model of institution-based clinics was no more viable than it would be to privately fund what would amount to national reproductive health care.

Neither independent nor institutional clinics provided an adequate solution to the problem of ensuring that all American women had access to contraception. Independent clinics were too expensive, and they could not cover areas with low population density. While institutional clinics were also usually located in cities, it was only through existing hospital and public health institutions that birth control activists could hope to reach women outside of urban centers. But these institutions did not value birth control services enough to support them financially. Birth control activists and the institutions they targeted were too far apart in the 1920s and 1930s to form a public-private partnership that might have made contraceptives far more available than the best efforts of five hundred individual clinics could do.

TWO

Inside the Birth Control Clinic

The twentieth-century reproductive rights movement was founded with Margaret Sanger's 1920 call to arms: "No woman can call herself free who does not own and control her body. No woman can call herself free until she can choose consciously whether she will or will not be a mother."[1] But if birth control activists believed in the right of all women to contraceptive information, their practical campaign to provide that information fell short of that ideal. When catchphrases were turned into clinic programs, the class-based traditions of charitable reform took over, in part to avoid controversy and criticism, but also because activists could not conceive of it any other way.

Birth control offered liberating freedoms to women who used it: increased leisure time, the ability to work after marriage, improved health, and a longer life span, but its adherents rarely linked it with new roles for men and women. Instead, they sought to enable working-class families to ape middle-class gender roles: a stay-at-home mother and a bread-earning father. Their clinics excluded single women, pregnant women, and many who wanted contraceptives for the wrong reasons. Most clinics also refused service to wealthy women, who they thought should consult private physicians. Some clinics would not aid a woman until she already had a certain number of children, while others would only accept women who were referred by a social worker, doctor, or clergyman. The modern notion of a Planned Parenthood clinic, open to any woman for advice, developed over time. In the 1920s and 1930s it was still distant. Choices were narrower then: abstinence, withdrawal, or an assortment of over-the-counter or mail-order products—rubber goods, jellies, ointments, and douches of sometimes dubious efficacy. The birth control clinic was a new option, treating only a small percentage even as the idea of birth control was taking root in the consciousness of American women.

Birth control clinics were created to address working-class mothers' problems as defined by the activists, and these definitions were both perceptive and biased. Activists operated on the assumption that working-class women wanted fewer children, and that they did not seek full-time outside employment. Activists knew that frequent childbearing compromised the health of mothers, strained marriages, and drained family incomes. They saw that the poor used less effective means of contraception than the wealthy and middle class and believed that the poor were ignorant of how both conception and contraception worked. Activists recognized that failing to avoid pregnancy, poor women would attempt abortion, an often ineffective and dangerous practice. Finally, birth control advocates believed that working-class women, not their husbands, should make decisions about reproduction.

Activists developed birth control clinics to provide cheap and effective contraceptives to those who would use them to improve their marriage and family life. Clinics offered married working-class women low-cost access to the same high-quality contraceptives used by middle-class women. Similar to tuberculosis clinics or well-baby clinics, birth control clinics promised tangible benefits to working-class families, including reduced maternal and infant mortality, higher standards of living, better health, and happier marriages. Birth control might also empower working-class men and women, but clinics downplayed such feminist or socialist agendas, instead arguing that any woman's most important role was being a wife and mother. Far from Sanger's demand that no woman be left in ignorance of birth control, many birth control clinic policies were designed not to make contraceptives available to *all* women, but to insure that *certain* women were able to get them.

Birth control activists selected the patients they wanted from a wide spectrum. The clinic's patients, described in newspaper articles, annual reports, and publicity brochures, put a carefully selected face on the birth control movement, one designed to attract the least opposition possible while still fulfilling a need. The "perfect patient" was a white married woman, who already had several children. Too poor to afford a private physician, she had some medical or eugenic reason to postpone additional children. It is also instructive to note what she was not. She was not obviously foreign, she was not portrayed as an immigrant, a Catholic, or an African American—not the kind of woman that nativists and eugenicists wanted to exclude from entering the United States. She also was not "unfit"—she might be underprivileged, but she was not the kind of depraved working-class woman whose intellect was as suspect as her morals. Carrie Buck, the famed poster child for forced sterilization, was not the kind of woman that the clinics wanted. Instead, the "perfect patient" was smart enough to use birth control to save her marriage, improve her health and that of her existing children, while insuring a chance of economic independence for her family. Multiplied in clinics across the nation, she served to improve American society, one diaphragm at a time.

Getting In: Admission Requirements at the Clinic

The image of the "perfect patient" answered critics who linked birth control with abortion, extramarital sex, immorality, selfish "new women," and quackery. By publicizing descriptions of patients whose need for contraceptives was so eminently reasonable, clinics created a loose consensus about the conditions under which any woman might legitimately postpone having children. During the boom years of the 1920s, birth control rhetoric was confined to poor women, but with the onset of the Great Depression, it took on a more universal appeal. Businesses failed, the economy shrank, and millions of savings accounts were swept away in bank failures. Unemployment, once a concern only for the poor, became the wolf at every door. By March 1933, some thirteen million were out of work, roughly 25 percent of the workforce. Many more people had been reduced to part-time or intermittent jobs. In difficult conditions like these, any woman, no matter what her social status, might consider delaying childbirth until things improved. Activists argued that women should space their babies at least two years apart to insure the mother's health, a rationale first applied to working-class women, but later directed towards all women. Ideas about child spacing, first discussed in the context of impoverished families, were gradually absorbed by the general public, even if they used private physicians for their own care. In this way, clinics served a public function broader than could be achieved by treating just those patients.[2]

Patients came to birth control clinics by way of referrals from doctors, hospitals, social workers, and clergymen, from friends, family, and other patients, and from the clinic's outreach and publicity efforts. No matter what brought them to the clinic, potential patients were interviewed to determine whether they would be accepted. Marjorie Prevost wrote of the BCCRB's liberal policy: "No patient is turned away from here if it is humanly possible to accept her, and if she is refused, it is due to the fact that she requires termination or it is *absolutely impossible* to find any health reason after the most careful and meticulous of examinations by the Doctor and a conference on the part of myself and the Doctor."[3] Only 13 percent of the women who consulted the bureau *were* turned away; the reasons ranged from a lack of a medical cause (a New York State law), to pregnancy, or the discovery of cancer or another medical condition.[4] Few clinics kept statistics on those they turned away, but the numbers were always highest in the clinic's first years. Clinic activists credited this to the awareness of their abortion policy, which "travels very quickly by word of mouth." In Los Angeles, the percentage of women turned away declined dramatically, from 14 percent in 1925 to only 3 percent by 1928.[5] By 1939, the BCFA reported that a similar 3 percent (of almost fifty thousand patients) were refused entry. Most rejected patients were already pregnant, but did not know it. Other common reasons were that the patient was not currently married or living with her husband, or that she made too much money.[6] By the late 1930s, prospective patients were more familiar with admission policies and knew if they would be accepted.

From the start, clinics excluded men from their programs. While it seems natural to us today, there was no real scientific reason why men could not have been responsible for contraception, or that the couple might have been the "patient," not just the woman. The most widely used methods of contraception, withdrawal and the condom, were male-controlled or required male cooperation. But this reality was one that birth control activists sought to change, both by pushing for woman-controlled contraceptives and designing their clinics (and by extension the birth control movement) as female spaces. Very few clinics prescribed condoms, though they were an inexpensive and effective method when used conscientiously. Clinics occasionally prescribed them for women who had failed using diaphragms or spermicidal jellies, but it was always a last resort, when the preferred options had been tried.[7] Birth control activists firmly believed that men could not be trusted in this matter, and saw traditional measures like withdrawal, rhythm, and the condom as flawed.[8] Working-class men made easy scapegoats for middle-class reformers who blamed them for failing to support existing children and irresponsibly insisting upon gratifying their sexual desires without care for their wives' desires or the risk of increasing their family. They also blamed working-class men for a variety of character flaws (drunkenness, violence, criminality) that damaged their families. One example of such characterizations comes from Arizona, where a BCCRB field worker reported: "The father is impossible—45 and drinks all the time. The minute he gets his relief money he begins drinking it up before he gets home—at times the authorities turn a deaf ear and a blind eye to him for if he gets arrested his money will cease and the children will starve. The day I was there he had just been released from jail after a fight in which a man was killed."[9]

At the Little Rock clinic, worker Hilda Cornish Coates referred to the patients' husbands as "beasts."[10] In the feminized space of the clinic, patients' descriptions of overweening, drunken husbands, in and out of prison, unemployed, or abusive were met with sympathy *and* a diaphragm. The underlying philosophy at the clinic sought to separate working-class women from solidarity with their men, in favor of an unequal sisterhood with the clinic activists.

Birth control clinics operated in a society where many opposed their work. They needed to blunt the criticisms of their opponents, fair or unfair, and portray their work in the most positive light possible. One way to accomplish this was to exclude some groups of women, and in doing so defend themselves from charges that they fostered immorality, provided abortion services, or offered the dreaded "birth control on demand." Drawing a line around what birth control activists thought the public would accept and support, admission policies manifested the activists' efforts to remain "respectable." Crossing that line—the placement of which varied over the course of time and with the changing beliefs of clinic activists—threatened the clinic's place in society, its ability to fund-raise, or even to operate legally. While some clinics were more likely than others to bend a rule here or there, no clinics regularly challenged the following array of beliefs and restrictions.

A key moral argument against contraception was that it tempted the unmarried to have sex because it removed the consequences of their trysts. Birth control clinics were accused of pandering to short-haired college girls, spreading their propaganda in high schools, and mailing their pamphlets to anyone who asked, regardless of their marital status. To combat these accusations, and in many cases to comply with state laws on contraception, birth control clinics refused to admit unmarried women. Critics demanded to know what proofs the clinics secured from their patients to assure that they were in fact married, intimating that the clinics condoned free love and promiscuity.[11]

Despite clinics' protests, opponents' suspicions lingered, and with good reason. How carefully did the clinics enforce their policies? What did they do about women who were about to be married? In these instances and others, clinics erred on the side of liberality. While clinics rejected women who admitted being single, there is no evidence that they investigated their patients' stories. This is not to say that clinic workers simply winked and let a series of "Mrs. Smiths" walk through the door, but it seems clear that a determined single woman could lie her way into a clinic. In one documented instance, an unmarried police decoy was admitted to a clinic, made it through the screening process, and would have been fitted for a diaphragm but left before the doctor could see her.[12] One way clinics tried to verify the identities of their patients was to require referrals from a social worker, doctor, or priest. This practice spread responsibility over a larger group, offering the clinic protection from the accusation that it accepted patients willy-nilly.

If clinics would not accept unmarried women, how would women about to be married get information? The answer at about seventy clinics, by the end of the 1930s, was to institute a service for engaged couples. Always a tiny minority of the patients (1.3 percent in 1937, or 400 of 30,000 patients), this service reflected a commitment to the idea of "child spacing," where a woman intentionally planned her children over the course of her marriage. The typical patient in the 1920s already had children, often in quick succession, and sought aid to *stop* reproduction, not slow it. By the 1930s, activists were seeing newlyweds who wanted to delay their first child until they were ready, and then space out future births to give the mother time to recover and build up resources. In order to accomplish this, it was critical that newlyweds get information.[13] Clinics presented a rosy view of how child spacing could improve family life: "The joy of motherhood became a reality when the patients were able to rest and recuperate between pregnancies, and when the planning of an addition to the family was a matter of mutual desire and consultation between husband and wife. Our patients are all beset by economic difficulties, but the love of a mother and a father for a wanted child make a happy home possible for more and more of these families each year."[14]

To protect themselves from the morally suspect practice of advising the unmarried, clinics employed a number of different strategies. Some, like the CMHA, required that an engaged patient provide written verification of her upcoming wedding from her minister. Cleveland was unique in that it offered sex education sessions to the wife during regular clinic hours, but also to husbands at evening lectures that explained female anatomy and contraception.[15] Many clinics offered premarital advice on sex and birth control but stopped short of prescribing a contraceptive until after the wedding, on the assumption that until then the patient would remain a virgin. Clinics sometimes prescribed condoms for the first few weeks, scheduling a diaphragm fitting only after marital sex had occurred.

Despite the appeal of child spacing, only a minority of clinics dared to offer premarital advice to their patients. The majority were somewhat uncomfortable with promoting the notion that birth control resulted in smaller families. In a 1936 survey of fifty-one clinics, only 30 percent of respondents thought clinics should see premarital patients, and only 53 percent thought that newlyweds should be treated. Some independent, settlement, and hospital-based clinics even refused to admit women who were childless, and a few required that a patient have two or more children (e.g., Indianapolis Maternal Health Center and the City Park Chapel in Brooklyn, New York). Still other clinics stiffened their normal requirements if the patient was childless, imposing a health requirement that they did not ask of a patient who was already a mother (e.g., the New York City Mothers' Committee settlement clinics and the Bethlehem Maternal Health Center in Pennsylvania).[16]

Most birth control activists saw their work as ameliorative rather than preventive. They felt most comfortable treating the "typical patient," defined as an overburdened mother of many children. They were far less sanguine when counseling a young childless woman, who might use her freedom to pursue paid labor after marriage. Most activists did not see themselves in the business of helping women avoid motherhood completely, unless there were compelling reasons for doing so. Instead, they believed that birth control would enable women to become better mothers. Clinics were proud of patients who bore a "planned" child, confirming their belief that women wanted children; they just wanted control over the timing.[17]

Abortion was exceptionally important to clinic founders. There was a great deal of confusion in the public mind between abortion and contraception. In keeping with their views on motherhood and maternity, most activists opposed abortion on principle, though there were compelling political reasons to do so as well. Birth control clinics shied from the issue, refusing to see pregnant women because by that time, contraceptive advice was too late. Offering any advice to pregnant women put a clinic at risk. If the woman later got an illegal abortion or suffered a miscarriage, the clinic would be suspected. From the earliest clinic in Brownsville, Brooklyn, activists separated birth control from abortion. In the flyer Sanger posted on Brooklyn streets in 1916, she exhorted "Do not kill, do not take life, but prevent."[18] The truth was that birth control and abortion were not so neatly compartmentalized in the minds of patients, doctors, or opponents of birth control as they were at the birth control clinic, where this artificial division was maintained as a defense mechanism.

The women who came to the clinics often did not know whether they were pregnant or not. In many cases, it was the fear of pregnancy that drove a woman to finally seek help. Such women were anxious and wanted to be seen immediately. Especially in the 1920s, some patients hoped to secure an abortion. Clinic staff did not share the patient's urgency, often asking women to return a few weeks later, once they were certain that they were *not* pregnant. By the 1930s, clinics began offering Ascheim-Zondek tests to accurately determine pregnancy. Those found to be pregnant were rejected, though they were advised to return after the baby was born. Half the women who came to one clinic certain that they were pregnant were *not.* The "A-Z test" was expensive and usually reserved either for paying patients, "desperate" cases where activists feared that the patient might do something drastic, or in cases when the mother's health would be endangered by pregnancy.[19]

While it was legal for a birth control clinic physician to refer patients for therapeutic abortions, very few did so. Most clinics that did provide abortions were in hospitals, where the procedure could be performed legally. These referrals, like those made by any private physician, were routed through a special panel empowered to evaluate the health risk of the pregnancy to the patient. This system of review absolved the clinic or doctor from responsibility. Referrals to private physicians were also legal, but the lack of oversight made the practice suspect. While it is impossible to know how often clinic workers referred patients for therapeutic abortions, the lack of evidence and reaction to the few instances found suggests that while exceptions may have been made in "extraordinary" cases, it was probably not a common occurrence. Birth control activists worked hard to separate abortion from birth control.[20] They also had no guarantee that the hospital or private physician would agree to actually perform the abortion. In the only instance I found of such a request, the BCCRB found its referral summarily rejected because the hospital did not agree there was a viable medical reason.[21]

In the voluminous Sanger papers, there are only scattered references to abortion referrals at clinics. This could reflect an unwillingness to document the event, but more likely it is a reflection of the rarity of the occurrence. Of particular interest is a 1927 report by the new ABCL executive secretary, Penelope B. Parker Huse, who found that Sanger's personal secretary, Anna Lifshiz, took it upon herself to refer "especially sad cases" to physicians for abortions. Huse strenuously opposed the policy, but Lifshiz remarked that it "had always been done." Huse "made a fixed rule that under no circumstances should anyone be helped to an abortion through contact with this office." Lifshiz left the ABCL shortly afterwards, but there is no evidence to suggest that she did so under duress; she remained Sanger's loyal follower for years.[22] No other reports were found of similar behavior until 1932, when the BCCRB's executive secretary Marjorie Prevost referred an unmarried healthy woman to a private physician for an abortion. In this case the patient's fiancé had abandoned her when he learned she was pregnant. The abortion was performed by an outside physician, and when Prevost reported the deed to Sanger she assured, "I immediately saw that she was of the class where you and I felt an exception could be made." Exception or not, Prevost was cautious, noting "I have been exceedingly careful, did not even write Dr. Siegal's address for her but had her do it herself on a piece of blank paper." Sanger's response warned, "It must be understood that whatever you do is on your own personal responsibility and not authorized by the Clinic. These are the hardest cases that we have to contend with, but we must safe-guard our work and those who stand behind us, such as our Advisory Council."[23] Despite Sanger's reprimand, Prevost was not disciplined. In 1942, Olga Willett, a new staff member, was also discovered referring patients for abortion. Reprimanded and transferred away from the reception desk, Sanger supported the action but wrote to the clinic supervisor, "Don't be too hard on her humanitarian spirit. It was not graft or for gain—not good for our Bureau but really heart rendering to interview women and our hands are tied. I'd be the last to throw a stone. Discipline must be kept— So in the supply room she goes."[24]

The few abortion referrals uncovered at the BCCRB were made by the lay staff, not by its physicians. There is no indication that the BCCRB doctors ever provided an abortion, although by New York State law they were allowed to do so for therapeutic reasons. Instead, the BCCRB's physicians tried to avoid all contact with pregnant patients. Sanger's creation of an "overdue" clinic in 1933 made this more difficult, as she tasked medical director Hannah Stone to study patients with overdue periods. The women were examined and if they were pregnant, counseled to keep their baby. In staff meetings, doctors advised that pregnant patients be kept away from the clinic and wanted them tested at a hospital clinic or dispensary, not on clinic premises. "Overdue" patients waiting to be seen by Stone were segregated in a separate waiting room so as not to spook new patients. Activists thought that seeing a failed case would weaken confidence in the clinic method.[25]

Activists argued that using contraception reduced abortions, but critics believed that if her contraceptive failed, a woman would be more likely to seek abortion to rid herself of the unwanted pregnancy.[26] Failed cases worried activists, and they took preventive steps. In one case, that meant investigating a clinician when her patients had abnormally high failure rates. Failures also created ethical problems for the doctors and activists. It was logical that if a patient merited birth control advice for health reasons, she ought to also merit a therapeutic abortion if her contraceptive failed. But few doctors were willing to act on that connection. Among themselves at least, one doctor argued that they should be willing to provide abortions to patients who became pregnant while participating in BCCRB contraceptive tests, but no action was taken on this proposal.[27]

I have discovered only one instance of a clinic doctor performing an abortion for a patient. The incident was revealed only because the clinic's staff disapproved and complained to Margaret Sanger, who was on the clinic's board. At the Tucson Mother's Health Clinic, a doctor induced an abortion for a critically ill patient, most likely a situation in which a therapeutic abortion was legally justified. The clinic's nurse supported the deed, claiming, "The woman was at her death-bed and by a miracle she was saved." But shortly afterwards, word began to spread among patients, and the nurse learned that the doctor had begun performing abortions in her private office. The nurse, Emma Hensley, took immediate action, warning Sanger, "Knowing that it should never have been done through the Clinic . . . I have since refused to call her for any further services." Hensley feared that her volunteer doctors might quit for fear of being tarred as abortionists.[28] So while a clinic might look the other way in an instance where a woman's life was in danger, they were far less tolerant of abortions done routinely, clandestinely, or for profit.

Any estimation of the frequency of abortion referrals at birth control clinics is little more than educated guesswork given the paucity of references. It does appear that some clinics were willing to make the occasional "exception" to aid a particularly sympathetic patient. Perhaps other reformers were like Margaret Sanger, who, though publicly disavowing abortion, would overlook attempts by her employees to help specific patients. Sanger was most likely aware of Lifshiz's referrals in the 1920s, and was obviously told about Prevost and Willett's deeds. None of the women were fired. Sanger's response in the Tucson case, recorded by her secretary in the letter's margin was: "MS thot it as well to do nothing on this for the time being."[29] When it came to abortion referrals, Sanger's chief concern was to keep the clinic out of trouble, not to reject the deed itself. I have found no evidence of abortion referrals or the provision of abortion in the records of any other clinics and it would appear that the activists who led these clinics had little tolerance for abortion. I doubt that these activists supported increased access to abortion because it did not match their views on motherhood and women's roles in the family. Also, though accusations that they provided abortion were leveled at many birth control clinics, no confirmed case ever seems to have been prosecuted over the two-decade period in question. Pregnant women, for the most part, had no place at the clinic; they were symbols of failed efforts at contraception, and helping them risked a dangerous link to the still-illegal world of abortion.

The third group of women refused admission at birth control clinics consisted of those whose reasons were deemed inadequate. Birth control activists organized the reasons for contraception into three large categories: *medical indications:* life- or health-threatening illness that made future childbearing dangerous (e.g., tuberculosis or heart disease); *economic indications:* inadequate resources to support additional children; and *social indications:* usually inheritable diseases or dangerous social circumstances (spouse abuse, alcoholism, criminality, or mental illness).

Many clinics accepted patients from all groups, but a significant minority accepted patients only for medical reasons. In states like New York, this restriction was the state law; in other places it was self-imposed. The definition of a medical indication varied considerably from clinic to clinic. While hospital clinics tended toward a more restricted list of conditions, such as heart disease, tuberculosis, kidney disease, or gynecological abnormalities that either prevented a woman from carrying babies to term or threatened her life, others were less strict. Independent clinics, like the BCCRB, stretched medical indications to breaking by claiming "child spacing" was a medical cause for birth control. This meant that they could legally treat any woman who had given birth within the last few years.[30] Medical Director Hannah Stone argued that the law interfered with her rights as a physician to prevent illnesses. When she examined a mother who could afford no more children, but was not yet physically ill, the only option was to advise abstinence, which she believed ineffective and psychologically harmful. The result of obeying the law left patients to try dangerous or useless devices, which then failed them, resulting in abortions.[31]

Interpretation and enforcement varied not only from clinic to clinic, but even from doctor to doctor within a clinic. Hospital clinic admission policies were stricter than independent clinics.[32] Women also reported that male physicians in private practice were reluctant to prescribe contraceptives. These doctors saw themselves as moral advisors and believed that women should fill traditional roles in society. Doctors wanted to help women recover their health after pregnancy in order to bear *more* children. They were less inclined to help them to stop childbearing. They characterized contraceptive-seeking patients as selfish and irresponsible. In an example from 1929, a thirty-two-year-old newlywed in good health sought contraceptives from Sanger's BCCRB, from private physician Mary Halton, and from Dr. Robert Latou Dickinson. She failed in all three places, but the nature of her failure reflected the differences in the sites. At the Sanger clinic, she reported that the desk worker informed her that without a medical reason the doctor could not see her; instead she suggested an over-the-counter contraceptive jelly. At Halton's crowded office, the woman left before being seen because the other clientele were "a group with which she was unwilling to be identified." Dickinson met her, but reportedly said, "being well able to afford a baby there was every reason to start her family and that urgency existed because she was beyond thirty." Dickinson refused to take a fee but was not interested in *her* reasons for postponing a family; instead he tried to convince her that she was misguided. Patient letters confirm that many private doctors had the same reservations, believing that they were better placed than their patients to know when contraceptives should be employed.[33]

Birth control activists believed that the poor needed birth control clinics more than the middle class or wealthy. Where reasons were recorded, economic need drove most patients to clinics. Between 55 and 91 percent of patients claimed they came to the clinic because they could not afford another child.[34] If health reasons for birth control were subject to interpretation, economic reasons were even more nebulous. Activists had to determine how poor a patient should be to qualify for aid, considering variables such as cost of living, the clinic's budget, and the patient's own economic situation—the number of dependents in the household, the regularity of work, and other factors. Rather than set a firm income amount for admission, most clinics relied on vague appellations: "indigent," "patients who cannot afford a private physician," or those "on relief."[35]

A small minority of clinics did not consider economic need for admissions, rather seeking to treat a broad spectrum of women who paid on a sliding, income-based scale. Among the best known were Sanger's BCCRB and the IBCL's downtown clinic. The rationale was that fees from more affluent patients could subsidize services for the less fortunate. At the IBCL clinic, some patients paid fees as high as $7.50 for the service. Patients with lesser means paid reduced or no fees, and were treated at the league's settlement clinics. Illinois state law did not restrict contraceptive service to health reasons, so the IBCL could offer their services to women who simply preferred the clinic to a private physician. And their clinic competed directly with Chicago doctors. The IBCL did not offer poor women a free ride. They worked closely with social agencies to analyze need and insisted that the patients make some form of payment whenever possible, arguing that patients who paid something, even if it was not the full cost, better appreciated and cooperated with the service. Though such policies generated income for the clinic, few adopted them, possibly because they attracted criticism from physicians. Opposed to any form of medicine that took away patient dollars, doctors characterized the clinics that treated pay patients as "rackets" that sought to profit from birth control.[36]

Even clinics that treated only poor patients were criticized for stealing income from local medical practitioners. The clinics denied the charge, claiming that their patients could not afford doctors. Where they did take pay patients, clinics argued that these women had already rejected their family doctor's advice. Again, the doctor had not lost any viable practice. But much like their marriage requirement, most clinics did not investigate patients' income levels or their claims that their doctors refused to prescribe them a contraceptive.[37]

Opposition to providing birth control for economic reasons occasionally turned into a referendum on society's responsibility to the poor. With the increasing deprivation brought on by the Depression, Sanger and other birth control activists argued that spreading contraception among relief clients would save the public money. Catholic spokesman Father John A. Ryan rejected that argument, calling birth control a "superficial" reform that blamed the poor for their own poverty rather than encouraging them to fight for social justice and welfare. The birth control movement fought against opponents' characterizations of their patients as immoral shirkers who sought smaller families to have extra funds for cars, radios, and other luxuries. Activists continually put forth descriptions of their most miserable and pitiable patients as a contrast. Neither depiction was entirely accurate.[38]

Fearing criticism, many clinics required written referrals from their patients. In seeking a recommendation from a physician, nurse, social worker, or clergyman, the clinic ceded responsibility to investigate patients to other community groups. Activists assumed that the referring party knew the patient intimately. A social worker would have seen the family's income, home, and family situation; referring doctors or nurses knew the patient's health problems; the patient's clergyman knew her marriage or family situation better than a clinic worker. Seeking outside referrals also kept good relations with the local medical and social work community, though they made the patient's life more difficult, and may well have discouraged some from attending.

Many clinics were willing to discomfit the patient in order to maintain local goodwill. They feared the wrath of the local medical society, and created admissions policies that deferred to the private practitioner. They requested that a woman first consult with her private physician if she had one (though it doesn't appear that they verified whether or not that was done). The clinic's willingness to support the medical profession went only so far, however. All clinics were willing to offer advice to a woman whose family doctor refused her aid. While the policy ostensibly protected the clinic against medical opposition, it did not make them popular among physicians, who referred only about 10–15 percent of all patients to clinics.

The last category of acceptable reasons for birth control was the so-called social reason, the term under which both hereditary, eugenic, and troubled family situations were lumped. These included women with a family history of mental or physical defects but also more loosely described instances where it might not be advisable for a family to have more children. A husband's or wife's alcoholism, criminality, or abusiveness to their spouse might become potent reasons to limit children in a troubled home. Birth control clinics offered aid to the insane or "feebleminded," especially when cases of "defective" children were already born. These eugenic indications, among the most charged with class bias, will be treated more fully in chapter 4.

Despite all these restrictions, the vast majority of women who stepped inside a birth control clinic were accepted. Likely, most knew the clinic's policies before they approached. Those who did not meet the criteria, whether unmarried, healthy, or too wealthy, were left to continue whatever method they had been using, whether it was from a drug store, mail-order catalogs, private doctor, or a cooperative husband. Whether their efforts were as successful as those who attended the clinic cannot be determined with any certainty. Clinic records argue that they were not.[39]

Once Inside: Services at the Clinic

Now we turn to women admitted to the clinic. In the 1920s and 1930s, you could find birth control clinics in brownstone houses in immigrant neighborhoods, downtown high-rise office buildings, hospital outpatient departments, settlement houses, church community centers, and city halls. But despite the different buildings, admission policies, and sponsors, the basic procedure of providing contraceptive information was fairly standardized. The prospective patient, whether clutching a scribbled address or a printed referral slip, would have to look carefully to find the clinic, as most offered only discreet signs (so as not to offend the neighbors). Entering the clinic nervously, the woman might see several others seated in a neat and homey waiting room.[40] One might have small children playing at her feet, another, looking very young, might be accompanied by a new husband or fiancé. Some would appear calm, while others might be just as edgy as our imaginary woman.

A nurse or social worker at the front desk would confirm that the woman had found the right location, and begin the interview process. At some clinics, interviews were taken in the waiting area, while others offered the privacy of a separate room. The interviewer was generally of a higher social status and education level than the patient. Clinics hired trained social workers, but also relied on their board members, their daughters, friends, and other middle- to upper-class volunteers. Nurses were sometimes used at the front desk, but in some instances the "nurse" was merely a lay worker dressed in white.[41] Though the interviewer wanted to make the patient comfortable, the questions were intrusive. Who referred you to the clinic? What does your husband do for a living? Is he working at present? How much money does he make? Do you work, and if so how much money do you make? When was your last menstrual period? How many times have you been pregnant? How many children have you borne? How many are still alive? Are they normal? Have you had any abortions? Were the abortions induced or spontaneous? Were you born in this country? Was your husband? What is your ethnic background? Your husband's? What religion do you practice? Have you tried birth control methods before? If so, did they work? How often do you have sex? Do you enjoy it? If not, why not? Though the clinic interviewer may have sought to make the process feel like a conversation, her was job to gather information the clinic used to determine whether or not to admit the patient.[42]

But more went on at the initial clinic interview than questions and condescension. Clinic workers imparted a wealth of information to the patient about birth control, their own bodies, and the clinic's policies and procedures. The interviewer could also guide the woman to present her case in a way guaranteed to get accepted. As one patient described her BCCRB interview: "She asked why I desired the information regarding contraception and I told her it was only because my husband and I were in debt and economically could not afford another child. She explained to me that under the New York law a health reason was required. I told her I had no health reason I could think of. She said that the doctor would examine me and that she might possibly find something that would allow her to give me the information."[43] The lay interviewer held a lot of power in such situations—she could have refused the woman admittance based on her answers, but instead alerted the patient that she needed to alter her answers when she spoke to the doctor. Many interviewers explained the notion of child spacing to the patients, and in many instances this served as the "medical" reason to admit them.

At some larger clinics, this general instruction was offered to groups of women, as patient volume made one-on-one conversations impractical. At the BCCRB, nurses instructed patients in the "facts of anatomy and feminine hygiene" before they consulted with the doctor. Clinic workers found that many women had only a hazy understanding of their own bodies, despite already having several children. At some clinics, sex education lectures were arranged as promotions to attract new patients and publicize the clinic. Often held in the evening and using slides and occasionally three-dimensional models of reproductive systems, clinic staff taught women not only how reproduction took place, but the rationale behind the contraceptives they would employ.[44]

Patients saw the doctor next. This consultation was one-on-one, though nurses or other clinic workers might be present, especially if the doctor was male. The doctor conducted a gynecological and medical examination, went over the data recorded by the nurse or social worker, and determined which contraceptive method was best. For many of the patients, this was their first gynecological examination; for some it was one of only a few physical exams they would ever have. Understandably, many were nervous and uncomfortable and clinics took care to try to select physicians who would reassure the patient. As BCCRB supervisor Elizabeth Arnold described the exams: "If you want to do it right, it takes a lot of time. Even if you teach the diaphragm. You can't do it in ten minutes. You have to spend time with this patient. You have to teach her. I said it takes 40 minutes—sometimes 30 minutes to 40 minutes to teach a patient the first time how to use a diaphragm. You have to take a history. You have to know background. Her attitudes, her needs. If she's afraid to touch herself."[45] The clinics were proud of the diagnostic service they offered, remarking that about half the patients examined were found to have previously undetected medical or gynecological conditions that required treatment.[46]

Ninety percent of clinic patients were prescribed the same contraceptive—the diaphragm in conjunction with a spermicidal jelly (of various chemical compositions). Because either method was reasonably effective on its own, the "clinic method" could be seen as overkill. The rates of success reached 90–95 percent, which justified its use, but it was expensive and not well loved. Women found it cumbersome and distasteful. It forced them to touch their sexual organs, it had to be cleaned and maintained between uses to prevent rubber deterioration. Spermicidal jelly could be greasy and stained clothing. In some rare instances it caused irritation to either the patient or her husband.[47] But perhaps the biggest adjustment was that using the clinic method put women in charge of contraceptive decisions. Unlike withdrawal, condoms, or periodic abstinence, the clinic method did not rely on the cooperation of a husband. While women often came to the clinic to get more control over their reproductive lives, they sometimes balked at the amount of work the method required. Some patients complained that it was "too complicated" or "sordid," and viewed the many rules as annoyance and bother. But for others, the method fostered great confidence.

Many patients found the diaphragm more trouble than it was worth. A 1935 CMHA study found that 40 to 45 percent of patients stopped using the diaphragm; a 1934 study, though, found that 85 to 90 percent stuck with it at the BCCRB and the Newark Maternal Health Clinic. The disparity between acceptance rates was probably due to patient selection and quality of the instruction, making it critical that clinic workers convince patients that the diaphragm was so far superior to traditional means of contraception that it was worth the bother. They also insisted that the patient had to shoulder the responsibility for contraception, no matter how difficult it might be. The clinic offered a kind of tough love to women used to passively acquiescing to their husband's control in matters of sex, or to the inevitable cycle of pregnancies when fertility was uncontrolled. If the method failed—and it did in about 10 percent of cases—clinics sought to learn the cause. Activists argued that it was not the method that failed, nor was it their instruction, but rather the patient's technique, a lack of dedication, or her failure to maintain the diaphragm or purchase adequate supplies of contraceptive jelly. Blaming the patient was easier than finding fault with the method, which the middle- and upper-class activists saw as scientific, advanced, and effective.[48]

The first visit to the clinic was critical. It often determined whether a patient accepted the method prescribed or slid back into older, less-effective habits. The initial medical examination and instruction determined the patient's confidence level. Under the supervision of the doctor, the patient practiced inserting and removing the diaphragm until the doctor thought that she was adept.[49] While clinic literature often claimed that the doctor would spend as much time as a patient needed, in reality the doctor's time was in demand. Faced with crowded waiting rooms, some clinics had nurses supervise the patient's practice. This allowed the doctor to see more patients. The clinic also sent home printed instructions for diaphragm care and use and welcomed patients to come back for a consultation if additional instruction was needed. Because securing the patient's acceptance of the diaphragm was so crucial, most clinics allowed their new patients to come to the clinic for an unlimited number of follow-up visits and consultations within the first year at no additional charge.[50]

Many clinics encouraged regular follow-up visits, to reinforce the instruction. Patients were instructed to return in a fortnight with their diaphragms in place. The doctor could then check the fit and the patient's technique. Clinic nurses inspected diaphragms each year for signs of decay, and the supply office refilled the patient's spermicidal jelly order at a price lower than the local drugstore offered. All these services aimed to keep in touch with the patient so that the clinic could observe her progress and maintain accurate records of success and failure. At annual checkups or refittings, doctors checked for any pelvic conditions that might affect the diaphragm's fit or effectiveness. When a patient did not return for the follow-up visits, clinic staff contacted them, either by mail or by sending a social worker to their home to encourage their return.[51]

While most clinics limited their work strictly to offering contraceptive information, others defined their work more broadly. Some clinics conducted contraceptive research to aid the birth control movement; others offered services like marriage counseling, infertility treatments, and in rare cases, sterilization. By their nature, it was the hospital-based clinic that offered the widest variety of medical services, including therapeutic abortions for some patients. By 1939, these added services were a very minor part of the clinic's work, though in the decades that followed they developed into the modern Planned Parenthood clinic, offering a wide range of sex education and gynecological services.[52]

Only a handful of clinics conducted in-house contraceptive research; chiefly these were the BCCRB, the Miami Mothers' Health Centers, and the CMHA clinic. Each clinic served thousands of patients each year, a large enough base to supply statistically relevant data. Initially, the goal was to prove that the diaphragms were effective. Later, clinics evaluated different designs and spermicidal formulas to rate brands. By the late 1930s, clinics tested foam powder contraceptives. But no other advances in contraceptive methods were made until the pill was first made available to clinics in the late 1950s.[53]

In the 1920s, activists used clinic research to defend the diaphragm's effectiveness for the working classes, a claim disputed by those who believed that people with lower incomes or intelligence needed simpler methods of contraception. Eugenicists believed that sterilization was a better choice for the "unfit" because they were too careless or ignorant to employ the clinic method properly. Clinicians battled these assertions, albeit sometimes brusquely, as when Dr. Bessie Moses asserted, "The Baltimore clinic has low grade morons who have been using the method for nine years successfully."[54] New York's Carol Nash argued that their chief problem with patients was not a lack of intelligence but a "defeatist attitude," and that the average relief patient, advised by a clinic, could practice contraception successfully.[55]

By the 1930s, clinicians turned toward testing and developing simpler and cheaper forms of contraceptives. The BCCRB became a clearinghouse for data on spermicides and diaphragms, sharing their findings with other clinics. In the late 1920s and early 1930s, Sanger hired chemist Helen Holt to conduct laboratory studies on the chemical content of commercial spermicides, and then followed up that work with clinical tests at the BCCRB. To no one's surprise, Holt found that fully half the spermicides available were ineffective, while those recommended by the clinic (based on lactic acid jelly) were, in fact, most effective and least irritating. By 1936, the BCCRB codified its tests by creating "white" and "black" lists of branded contraceptives to guide physicians and clinics in selecting products.[56]

At Lydia deVilbiss's three Florida clinics, "foam powder," a new contraceptive method, was pioneered and developed, using patients as research material. It was a spermicidal powder that was shaken onto a sponge, moistened and squeezed until it foamed, and then inserted in the vagina. Cheaper than the rubber diaphragm, the foam powder and sponge method did not need expert fitting, which meant it could be dispensed by public health nurses instead of physicians. Available at clinics or druggists, foam powder offered activists a chance to spread birth control beyond the confines of the clinic. But the powder did not provide the elusive "magic pill" that Sanger and other birth control reformers sought. Clinical trials in Miami and in other American cities were generally positive, but British and Indian tests found the powder irritating. While it remained in use in some clinics, it never replaced the diaphragm as the contraceptive of choice.[57]

Not all contraceptive research sought to discover new methods. In Cleveland, researchers sought to test the "rhythm" method. They set up separate clinic hours for this experiment, taking detailed records from volunteer patients to determine when ovulation took place, and if any days within the menstrual cycle could be considered "safe." In 1936, the Brush Foundation funded this study and another one in Puerto Rico, which gathered similar information in an effort to develop an effective Catholic-sanctioned contraceptive method.[58]

Because these three clinics engaged in research, the vast majority of other clinics did not need to. The results of their studies were distributed through journals like the *BCR* and the *JOC* and at conferences. Most clinics simply adopted the recommended methods, reluctant to "experiment" on their patients. Research clinics alone had to grapple with the problem of testing new formulations or methods that might be *more* likely to fail than the accepted clinic method. But without those tests, no advances in contraceptive technology could be made. With mainstream science uninterested in the field, research and testing had to be done by activists in their clinics. Each clinic had to balance their patients' needs against the movement's needs. At research clinics, activists needed to pick the best patients to participate in the research trials. In the early years, the BCCRB tests were conducted on groups of one hundred women who were prescribed the same combination of spermicidal jelly and diaphragm. If four patients became pregnant, the method was rejected as ineffective, for activists wanted a success rate of 97 percent or better.[59] When volunteers in Cleveland were recruited for the rhythm study, they joined with a full understanding that they risked a pregnancy.[60] There is no indication that patients were encouraged or coerced to participate, either by financial inducements or reduced cost of supplies or exams.

Most clinics had to decide which patient services they would offer. Clinic activists learned that providing birth control was only part of the solution to working-class women's dilemmas. Many had marital problems or lacked basic knowledge of childcare, sex, or their own bodies; others suffered sexual phobias brought on by fears of incessant childbearing, or serious health problems that went beyond what could be addressed at a contraceptive clinic.

Clinic workers found that even when the fear of pregnancy was removed, many working-class women were still unfulfilled by or resistant to sex. A number of clinics offered marriage counseling sessions, where activists advised men and women on reasonable sexual expectations. At the CMHA clinic, the husband and wife were interviewed separately and offered "tactful counsel." In 1933, the BCCRB added a special "Marriage Consultation" service, run by Hannah Stone and her physician husband Abraham. Offered to married and engaged couples on a weekly basis, the Stones counseled couples on sex, contraception, and marriage for an annual fee of five dollars. From the sessions, the Stones published *A Marriage Manual: A Practical Guide Book to Sex and Marriage*, in 1935. The Stones aimed to end the marital maladjustments generated by the fear of pregnancy. Hannah Stone believed such fears hung "like the sword of Damocles over every sex intimacy," and were "the greatest deterrent to a normal sex-expression," as well as "a fertile source of much discord." Chicago doctor Rachelle Yarros founded the IBCL's sex education program in 1932, which offered lectures to churches, factories, and settlement houses. She exhorted: "We must teach them that sex gratification in moderation plays a very important part in life apart from the rearing of a family, because it is necessary to intimacy and tender affection between the husband and wife."[61]

A few birth control clinics offered infertility services by the end of the 1930s, arguing that their knowledge of contraception could and would be used to help the infertile. This was in keeping with the argument that parents should determine when they were ready for children. When faced with the occasional patient desperate to *have* a child, these clinics tried to help. Doing so deflated critics who accused the clinics of being anti-baby. Few clinics had any expertise in fertility work, and most often the service was added after 1940, but at least one, the Cincinnati Committee on Maternal Health, accepted infertility patients at its founding in 1929.[62] Part of the slow shift from "birth control" to "planned parenthood," infertility clinics were built on the overall plan of spaced children and general reproductive health care.

Clinics avoided sterilization almost as much as they did abortion services. Activists believed that there was a role for sterilization in the range of available reproductive services, but in almost every case, they did not want to be directly involved. As Sanger put it in 1932, "It has been my own experience that it is best to keep the two movements separate. There are many ardent supporters of birth control who do not believe in sterilization at all, and who would prefer segregation to sterilization for the feeble minded."[63] Sterilization was seen as appropriate in instances where a woman, due to health or other condition, would *never* be able to withstand a pregnancy. In these cases birth control, with its small, yet real risk of failure, was not enough. Sterilization was not advisable when a woman might want to become pregnant later or when her medical condition could improve. Sterilization was reserved for instances of physical or mental impairment, for women who would never be able to properly take on the responsibility of motherhood.[64]

Only a handful of clinics provided sterilization. Again, hospital clinics were the most likely to do so. At the Colorado General Hospital, sterilization was recommended for "the more irresponsible class of women." Chicago's Mandel Clinic at the Michael Reese Hospital also offered sterilization to its patients, reporting that because of it, their patient totals decreased from 102 to 58. Some women preferred sterilization to the continued use of contraception, finding it easier and cheaper. Most independent clinics, like the Los Angeles Mothers' Clinic, treated requests for sterilization by referring the woman to a hospital or physician for evaluation and treatment.[65]

Two clinics did offer sterilizations, the Florida Mother's Health Clinics, run by Dr. Lydia deVilbiss, and Dr. Muriel Cass's Palama Settlement in Honolulu. In both cases, sterilizations were performed predominately on nonwhite patients and there are indications that the patients may either have been pressured or deceived. The paucity of documentary evidence from either clinic complicates efforts at any analysis. DeVilbiss reported having advised and performed almost one hundred sterilizations in 1937, most on the husbands of her patients. Though she claimed to have explained the procedure clearly and secured consent, she privately admitted that the written release never mentioned the word sterilization. DeVilbiss argued that sterilization was the right choice for patients with "feeble-minded, diseased and psychopathic personalities, also those with gross pathology who should never procreate children."[66] At the Palama Settlement in Honolulu, Dr. Muriel Cass, described as "fearless and resolute," was responsible for more than eight hundred sterilizations, almost six hundred of which were performed on men at her clinic's office. Because the procedure for women was more complicated, the women were sterilized at local hospitals. The Palama clinic treated mostly Filipino and Puerto Rican patients, often referred by federal relief programs. Cass advised sterilization for these patients as the "only real answer" to contraception's drawbacks. She sterilized patients either for physical or mental disabilities that, in her mind, made contraceptive use impractical. Though the Palama Settlement claimed the operations were performed at "the request of both parties involved, and after careful investigation," it appears that inducements, in the form of work relief positions may have been linked to cooperation. More research needs to be done on the issue of sterilization at clinics, but the few sources available indicate that these two clinics were anomalies.[67]

Birth control clinic services reinforced the maternalist ideology of the clinics' activists. They were geared to help the working-class wife meet traditional ideas of motherhood and companionate marriage. The information that the clinics provided was supposed to help patients make their marriages work, help them to have regular and enjoyable sex with their husbands, and to take care of a family whose size matched their income. While the tool of birth control could be used by the patients to attain independence from husbands or freedom from family burdens, or even the ability to embark on a career, the impetus had to come from the patient. The clinic would not encourage it.

By restricting their services narrowly to birth control, the majority of clinics were content to focus on one aspect of women's health and welfare separated from larger social, political, or economic reform movements. Birth control activists argued that their patients were ignorant, but did not work with educational charities to school them; they described their patients' miserable poverty, but did not ally with reforms to restructure American society, improve urban housing, or expand job programs for the unemployed. They worked with chronically ill patients, but did not join movements for national health coverage. Birth control was an ameliorative reform; its adherents accepted the inequities of society and sought to work around them by helping to create smaller families. Some birth control activists had a broader outlook, especially at settlement clinics, but they did not use the birth control movement as a platform for arguing those larger social issues. Perhaps many of them did not share these goals. Like the neo-Malthusians of England, some American activists surely believed that workers who wanted to better their lot needed to adapt their lives to the inequities of capitalist society rather than try to change it. Others may have felt that arguing the feminist or socialist rationales for birth control could alienate potential supporters, especially donors, doctors, or politicians. But by limiting their interest in the working class to such narrowly defined health and economic issues, birth control activists failed to gather a larger constituency of women bent on securing advancement and liberation. They failed to make connections with other groups working for social justice because activists reasoned that a narrow focus strengthened their hand when dealing with the medical men and public health officers they hoped would take charge of the movement.

THREE

Clinic Activists

Clinics depended on a working relationship with physicians, but at its core, birth control was a lay movement, dominated by women without medical training. They were the wives of professional men, amateur social workers, and local philanthropists who created privately funded medical services for poor women, in a movement that promoted the kind of "socialized medicine" that organized medicine despised.

By the 1939 birth of the BCFA, women had ceded control over the national movement to male doctors and public health experts. They hoped to gain greater respectability, increased funding, and the integration of birth control in public health programs. As argued first by Linda Gordon in her 1976 book, *Woman's Body, Woman's Right*, and by Carole McCann in 1994's *Birth Control Politics in the United States*, the new organization marginalized women's work and experience in a shift towards "planned parenthood," a movement that relied on experts and paid professional staff.[1] Even Margaret Sanger, birth control's founder and inspiration, was not immune. When the BCFA emerged from the internecine squabbles of the ABCL and BCCRB, Sanger became "honorary president," allowing the BCFA to use her name but ceding all power. These new national leaders denigrated their forebears, characterizing the movement of the 1920s and 1930s as emotional, woman-focused, and out of touch with modern science.[2] Gordon and McCann's interpretations of the national movement are cogent, but they do not tell the whole story. At the local level, in the clinics, lay women retained both practical and financial control well into the 1940s. These organizations did not follow the national lead and hire paid professionals because their work focused on the delivery of services, not on lobbying or public relations. The power struggles between "Sangerist" women and organization men, depicted in McCann's work, did not happen at the local level. Professional men were not attracted to the work of local leagues or clinics and the provision of birth control services remained very much in the realm of women. While medical men advised clinics, and in some cases worked at them, they did not devote the excessive amounts of time or money needed to operate the clinics.

This chapter explores the relations between clinic activists, both lay and medical—a story as much about gender as it is about professionalization. Most lay activists were women and most doctors associated with clinics were men. The women were responsible for clinic administration, clerical work, fund-raising, staff hiring and supervision, and publicity. Men limited their association to offering advice, either medical, legal, or financial, and taking on paid clinical positions. Aside from clinicians, they were not involved in day-to-day clinic operation. This is wholly understandable, as birth control was seen as a woman's issue. Only the medical aspects of the work attracted the interest of men.

Lay Activists: Women and Men

Lay women drove the creation and expansion of birth control clinics, especially before 1937, when public health clinics began to be organized in greater numbers. While medical support was needed to reduce opposition to clinics, organizing a successful league or clinic was almost impossible without the help of lay women. As Caroline Robinson wrote in 1930, the clinic organizer's first step was to locate "every wealthy woman and every active woman volunteer in charity" and persuade her to sponsor the clinic because "these women represented both millions in money and also nearly every philanthropy in town."[3] Once convinced to work for birth control, society women's extensive contacts helped ally the clinic with social work and civic organizations. This helped secure patient referrals and promote a respectable face for the clinic. Clinic organizers also worked with the national organizations, attending conferences and networking with other activists. In each city, a clinic needed at least one (and preferably more than one) dedicated woman to rally support, bring together funding, medical support, and patients, and keep the organization together when initial enthusiasm flagged.

Lay women took on the jobs that needed to be done each day to keep the clinic going. Most did not hire secretaries or staff to administer the clinics, but instead donated both their time and money to run the clinics on relatively small budgets. Their daily or weekly contact with the clinic, interviewing patients, driving them to and from appointments, and recording detailed medical records kept the clinic activists personally and emotionally engaged. This level of connectedness helped when lay activists went out to raise funds or promote the clinic—they could offer examples of cases and discuss the lives and predicaments of their patients.[4]

Many clinics were fully funded by the steady contributions of a handful of women. Larger-scale clinics were more expensive to operate, with paid medical and clerical staff and extended hours. Even in these large clinics, volunteers played a crucial role managing thousands of medical records and stocking a variety of contraceptive supplies. When the budgets outstripped the ability of lay-women contributors, clinics such as the BCCRB and CMHA turned to private foundations and expanded their circle of wealthy donors. When the IBCL faced this challenge, it used a different tactic, arranging with social institutions around the city to "adopt" a clinic and to raise the funds needed to operate it. Thus, while Sanger solicited grants for the BCCRB from the Rockefeller's Bureau of Social Hygiene, the Julius Rosenwald Fund, and wealthy individuals such as Doris Duke, George Eastman, and Robert Wood Johnson, in Illinois the league turned to settlement houses and women's charities. The Chicago Woman's Aid organization adopted the IBCL's Medical Center number 5, while Hull House supplied space, physicians, and staff for Medical Center number 6. The average clinic, much smaller in scale, could be supported with small but steady donations from a handful of women. Clinic budgets fluctuated depending on how they were structured. Some had to pay rent, others hired nurses and doctors. Depending on the number of paying patients, costs could rise dramatically as clinics had to stock diaphragms and contraceptive jellies. A small clinic with volunteer physicians that operated in donated space might have an annual budget of about $700; one that paid rent and some staff salaries might need $6,000 per year. The BCCRB's annual budget was between $30,000 and $40,000 in the 1930s, undoubtedly the highest in the nation.[5]

A clinic's lay founders also volunteered as staff. Their efforts were crucial to keeping the clinics growing, as they provided a more educated worker than the clinic could afford to hire. This also further strengthened the lay founders' hold over the clinic. All clinics, even large-scale ones such as the CMHA and BCCRB, supplemented their paid workers with volunteers who undertook administrative and clerical work such as filing, manning literature desks, and selling refills of contraceptive jelly. They also handled special research projects, such as compiling patient statistics for a research study or generating lists of delinquent patients for social workers to visit. Some clinics made distinctions between medical and lay tasks, but at the numerous smaller clinics lay women filled almost all the posts save those of physicians themselves. At the Pennsylvania Birth Control Federation, Dr. Clarence J. Gamble privately crowed, "Almost all the histories are being taken by volunteers, and I am allowed to dress some of them up in uniforms and let them pose as nurses."[6]

What kinds of women were attracted to birth control activism? For the most part, they were the "women of wealth and intelligence" that Sanger targeted in the aftermath of her Brownsville clinic prosecution.[7] Most were middle-aged, college-educated, married women with grown children. Experienced in community activism and charitable endeavors, they were former suffragists, members of the League of Women Voters, and active members of local Parent-Teacher Associations and school boards. The benefactors of playgrounds and libraries, they kept active in garden, literary, and bridge clubs. As socialist Caroline Nelson derided them in 1929, they were the "people who in the early days were our enemies, who were for birth control, but not for anarchistic law breakers."[8] In short, because of their wealth these women had the leisure time to devote to causes. A major part of Sanger's drive to mainstream birth control in the 1920s aimed at attracting these social "pillars," whose support could counteract suspicion. Activists courted respectable women in order to increase the movement's status. Few activists were newly married or unmarried. They had no ties to contraceptive manufacturers, or any obvious personal motivations for participating in the movement. Activists were not usually socialists or radicals (Margaret Sanger notwithstanding) who might tarnish the newly burnished reputation of the movement. These very early pioneers of the birth control movement, active between 1912 and 1920, did not establish clinics.[9] When Sanger selected the first ABCL Board of Directors, she sought married women, aged forty-five to fifty-five years old. She looked for the wives of prominent professional men—stockbrokers, Wall Street lawyers, physicians, journalists, and business executives.[10] Most had children, though none had more than four. Charlotte Hoffman Delafield, vice president of the ABCL, is a good example. The wife of Wall Street lawyer Lewis Delafield, she was married in 1885, when Sanger was but a six-year-old. Delafield had three grown children when she joined Sanger's campaign in 1917. Delafield's prominence counteracted Sanger's reputation as a radical and troublemaker. As Sanger put it: "By her very demeanor and looks—white-haired, a fragile countenance—you knew she could touch nothing that was not fine, and that she had the spiritual courage to stand by her idea and ideals in both her public and private life."[11]

Clinic founders came from a similar caste. Helen Graham Carpenter of the IBCL was the wife of Chicago business executive Benjamin Carpenter and was known throughout Chicago for her civic work. She was fifty-five years old, with four grown children, when the first IBCL clinic was opened in 1923. Carpenter was not a radical by any definition. She was the first director of the Girl Scouts in Chicago, deeply involved in the American Genealogical Association, and happened to be the IBCL's second president.[12]

Mary Blessing Nelson, associated with the Visiting Nurse and Child Welfare Association in Reading, Pennsylvania, and a member of the board of the Child Assistance League, founded the Reading clinic. Won over by one of Sanger's lectures in 1918, Blessing began working locally for birth control shortly thereafter. She did not rush out and found a clinic immediately, but carefully built support and then capitalized on public interest created by another series of birth control lectures. Nelson had been a suffragist and welfare activist, with some associations with local socialists. On Sanger's advice, Nelson tested Pennsylvania's strict anti-birth control laws in 1927, opening the Berks County Maternal Health Clinic only to find the law "a lifeless legality." Years later, Nelson admitted to Sanger that it was her visits to Reading that "gave to us poor scared souls the courage to go on with the fight."[13]

The women who founded birth control clinics in the 1920s had the confidence to champion a controversial topic; they did not fear ridicule or scorn. Many were introduced to the cause by Sanger herself, as she lectured across the country exhorting wealthy women to join the movement. By all accounts a magnetic speaker who inspired women to action, Sanger's birth control propaganda was new and appealing. Before she modernized the movement, contraception was tangled in moral arguments, lumped in with abortion, and associated with political radicals. It was tainted by feminist arguments and radical class-baiting. Sanger recast the movement in the mantle of maternal welfare, where her target audience felt comfortable and competent.

To gather supporters, activists needed to deflect critics who saw contraceptive use as selfish and immoral. Led by Sanger, activists contended that having fewer children allowed women to be better mothers. They believed that most women wanted children, just not as many and as quickly as nature brought them. Sanger posited that mothers were the best qualified to decide when to have children, as they knew their home conditions intimately and would make their decisions in the best interests of their existing children. This would invariably reduce the number of abortions and maternal and infant deaths. This popular argument appealed to club women and social workers; it dovetailed with their interest in the maternal and infant welfare movement. These progressive reformers had already spawned the Children's Bureau, milk stations, well-baby clinics, postpartum care and educational programs for mothers, as well as the promotion of breast-feeding. Birth control, pitched in terms of maternal welfare, fit neatly into such programs. It promised to reduce mortality rates by reducing at-risk pregnancies and offered social reformers a new avenue of reform while staying in the domestic sphere. Underlying Sanger's argument was the idea that working-class women would use their newfound leisure time to become better mothers, not to seek jobs or further education. This appealed to activists because it focused on women and the family without creating a politically active underclass willing to organize for social change.[14]

As the movement gathered momentum in the 1930s, the women attracted to it changed. They were younger and more likely to be in their childbearing years. As before, most were married, but often their husbands had not yet risen to the tops of their professions. Many were associated with the Junior League and organizations that supported kindergartens and playgrounds.[15] Older women were still founding clinics in the 1930s, but they were aided by women a generation younger. In Little Rock, Hilda Kahlert Cornish was fifty-four years old when she founded the Arkansas Eugenics Association in 1930. The mother of six, Cornish was married to a successful banker and was deeply involved in civic and welfare associations. An active PTA member, she founded playgrounds and worked with charitable organizations and the Community Chest. Named president of the Arkansas Federation of Women's Clubs, by the late 1920s Cornish was a key worker in flood relief efforts and was president of the Council of Social Agencies. In 1928, economic uncertainty and personal tragedy jolted Cornish out of this comfortable life; her husband committed suicide when his bank collapsed. Shortly afterwards, she turned to birth control as her primary charity. She had an "in" few others did; her oldest son was the Yale roommate of Margaret Sanger's son Stuart. Thus Cornish became one of

Sanger's most loyal lieutenants. The Arkansas Eugenics Association opened the Little Rock Birth Control Clinic in 1931, and Cornish ushered in a true second generation of birth control activists, securing the participation of her daughter, Hilda Cornish Coates, daughter-in-law Sylvia Allen Cornish, and their friends. Hilda Cornish Coates was a Bryn Mawr graduate, twenty-eight years old, with three children born in four short years of marriage. An active member of the Junior League, Coates recalled volunteering almost every day either with the league or the clinic. She accompanied clinic patients through their medical examinations and fittings (the Little Rock clinic used male physicians) and was a member of the board of governors. Coates also took personal advantage of her association with the clinic—she was fitted for a diaphragm in 1932, and bore no more children.[16]

The explosive growth of birth control activism was built on such networks of women—some linked by family, others by social contacts. Hilda Cornish Coates brought fellow Junior League member Mary Louise Boaz Hall to work at the Little Rock clinic. A Barnard graduate who had done missionary work in Asia, Hall was a restless young wife with one small son. She was experienced in social service and had already founded a nursery school before joining the Arkansas Eugenics Association. With her came her husband, Graham Roots Hall, a lawyer who worked with the Community Chest and YMCA, and his sister, Emily Hall Harder, the wife of a salesman. Louise Hall and Emily Harder volunteered at the reception desk and assisted the staff doctors. Another officer, Raida Cohn Pfeifer, the clinic's receptionist and executive committee and board of governors member, brought her mother-in-law Heloise Pfeifer, her mother, jewelry-store heiress Marcuse Stifft Cohn, her sister, Miriam, and her merchant brother-in-law Arthur Phillips onto the board.[17] In Cleveland, connections between activists were also based on family and business ties. In addition to Dorothy Brush, the initial CMHA board drew members from the Brush Foundation: Edna Brush Perkins, and her husband Dr. Roger Griswold Perkins, Rosalyn Weir, her husband William Weir, and Brush family lawyer, Jerome Fisher.[18] Many local birth control leagues were likewise tightly knit organizations of friends and family members.

This second generation of activists was more locally focused. They were less likely to have met Margaret Sanger or other national leaders, and instead relied on written communications with New York or Washington for information and support. No new leader of national prominence emerged from this generation of reformers to snatch the birth control torch from

Margaret Sanger or interpret birth control for a new generation. Early in the 1920s, Sanger jealously guarded her primacy in the movement, described by one co-worker as "number one, and there was no number two; she would let no one approach her that closely."[19]

But by the late 1930s, Sanger was not the dominating force that she had once been. Looking to retire from active work, she was casting about for a successor but found few candidates. Though she was still the public face of the movement, she no longer controlled it and had little power over local organizations.[20] Some leagues refused to affiliate with Sanger's ABCL, even after she resigned in 1928. Even when they did affiliate with national leagues, few local clinic heads sought national recognition or power. At the end of the 1930s, ABCL officers and board members were drawn from the same clique of prominent New York women that originally filled the seats in 1921. While Sanger brought in women from state clinics and leagues as regional chairs of the NCFLBC, she held power tightly, making them responsible for their states but not for determining the NCFLBC's legislative tactics. The clinic activists in the 1930s focused on alleviating conditions in their own cities. While they supported the larger national program, few contributed the requested dues to the ABCL; most were loathe to assist the NCFLBC to raise funds or lobby their supporters for fear of siphoning off funds from their own work. Some leagues were reluctant to publicize their clinics for fear of attracting opposition, prompting Sanger to deride them as "speak-easy clinics," useless to the majority of women who were unaware they existed.[21] The Nebraska Maternal Health League acknowledged the failing, reporting in 1936: "Many of our board feel that it is better to continue the good work we are doing than to stir up antagonisms. Perhaps as we grow older we will be less timid."[22]

The CMHA provides an extreme example. Its founders, Dorothy Hamilton Brush and Hortense Oliver Shepard, had seen the opposition that birth control could generate when they attended the 1921 ABCL Conference. Sanger and several associates were arrested at the meeting at the instigation of Catholic archbishop Patrick J. Hayes. Back in Cleveland, they worked cautiously and quietly for five years to gather support among older matrons. Keeping a low profile while lobbying individual Cleveland lawyers, doctors, and prominent members of society, they waited until 1928 to launch their first birth control clinic. They also avoided entanglements with national birth control organizations until 1942, viewing their work as a local charity rather than as a branch of the controversial national movement. This example would be repeated time and time again.[23]

Lay men who served at clinics were rare, usually the husbands, sons-in-law, brothers, or friends of the women activists. They often performed accounting or legal services for the clinic, but were peripheral to its daily work. Graham Roots Hall provides a typical example. Brought in by his wife, Hall was the legal advisor to the Little Rock clinic, investigating laws on contraception and negotiating contracts and legal agreements. Other men were treasurers or accountants, donating their time to audit the clinic's books or develop budget plans. Several clinics relied on men to negotiate deals with contraceptive manufacturers and suppliers, a role that J. Noah Slee, Sanger's second husband, relished at the BCCRB. But few lay men had more than a marginal connection to the clinic's daily operations, as officers, members of the executive committee, or administrative or clerical workers in the clinic. Instead they shied from the clinic premises. Most simply lent their prestigious names to clinic advisory councils, listed on letterheads and annual reports. Unlike their wives, these professional men had less time to devote to charitable enterprises and many did not think it appropriate to become deeply engaged in a reform movement that fostered emotional connections with working-class women. Thus, while prominent businessmen, doctors, and clergymen swelled the lists of Advisory Councils, Governing Bodies, and Clinic Committees, these bodies rarely, if ever, met and had no direct responsibility at the clinic.[24]

Eugenicists were a distinct subgroup of lay activists involved with the birth control movement, though one that followed the general pattern of limited direct involvement. Male eugenicists were often academics associated with university departments of genetics or social science. As members of an advisory board, male eugenicists provided clinics with scientific credentials, just as the names of wealthy women offered social cachet. Like physicians, eugenicists often did not believe that the patient should be the key decision maker in questions of contraception, but they supported more broadly defined admission rules than doctors. Lay activists could therefore pit eugenicists against doctors on their boards, using eugenicists to press for the expansion of the service to women with economic and social indications.[25]

At the BCCRB, Sanger used nationally prominent eugenicists like Edward Murray East, a Harvard biologist and geneticist who wrote extensively on the dangers facing the human race; Raymond Pearl, a statistician and geneticist at Johns Hopkins University; University of Wisconsin genetics professor Leon J. Cole; and former president of the University of Michigan, Clarence Cook Little, to back her position against medical critics. The BCCRB allowed eugenicists access to its patient records, in order to fuel studies on the impact of contraception. Pearl's studies on contraceptives supported the clinic activists' contentions that it was not race or heredity that led to large families, but a lack of access to contraceptives.[26] To them, women with husbands on relief, or who were alcoholic, abusive, or "feebleminded" were good candidates for birth control, and they provided an impressive body of work, no matter how flawed it appears today, supporting the hereditarian nature of these traits.[27]

Women played an important role in the eugenics movement, but not as its leaders. In part this is because we define eugenicists as those who made scientific arguments for practical efforts to increase the fitness of the general population. We do not generally refer to eugenicists as those men and women who accepted these arguments, funded eugenics efforts, or attended presentations, which is the way most women participated in the eugenics movement. Some women found work doing research for eugenicists, who often preferred them to men. Women who became involved with eugenics work often came from backgrounds similar to those of women attracted to birth control reform, but the two groups did not overlap much. Both were attracted to reform movements that bettered the lot of children, but a woman who put eugenics before birth control might focus on issues such as homes for handicapped children, work on welfare boards, or the regulation of child labor. We don't know enough about the average clinic activist's beliefs to know how eugenic thought played out in their birth control ideas. But there are rare instances of women who worked in both movements. Jean Gordon, a New Orleans activist, was known for her work with Milne Home, where "mentally deficient" patients were either sterilized or segregated. She opened the first birth control clinic in that city. The close connection between the CMHA and the Brush Foundation, which funded eugenic research, does not appear to have affected the workings of the clinic. In Augusta, Georgia, activist Nora Nixon, the executive director of University Hospital's Maternal Health Clinic, was a known sterilization proponent. As historian Edward Larson posits, women who found eugenics appealing may have harbored a deep-seated elitism and racism that prompted them to look fondly on more coercive methods of improving the population.[28]

Only a handful of lay men led clinics or birth control leagues. One, William Hazlett Upson, was the founding president of the Middlebury Maternal Health League in Vermont. Upson was best known for his short stories, which were serialized in the *Saturday Evening Post* and featured tractor salesman Alexander Botts. He was an active campaigner for aid to handicapped children as well as a local Republican politician. Upson argued the need to reduce the high levels of fertility among the "unfit," but he chose not to open a sterilization clinic or a traditional birth control clinic; rather, he created a referral service that linked willing doctors with patients who needed aid.[29]

The Lincoln Maternal Health Association was a rare league with predominantly male leadership. Unitarian minister Arthur L. Weatherly served as president, while dentist Frederick F. Teal was its vice president, and Thurl B. Strain, a banker, was its treasurer. Weatherly's social activism included the suffrage movement, the fight for workman's compensation, the founding of the Lincoln General Hospital, and the creation of a local Urban League branch. The only female officer was the chair, a position held by Nellie Sellers and Mabel Leverich Throop. The officers presided over a twenty-six-member board of directors (seventeen women and nine men) and a ten-member, all-male medical advisory board. But women, even in Lincoln, did the practical work that kept the clinic running—heading working committees dealing with operations, finance, and membership. They also supervised the female medical director. Even when men held top positions in organizations, the eight-member "Clinic Committee" was populated entirely by women. After Rev. Weatherly left the Lincoln League to become president of the Nebraska State League in 1940, a woman, Cornelia Frazier Putney, replaced him.[30]

Men also led a handful of state leagues. In addition to Weatherly in Nebraska, the Pennsylvania Birth Control Federation selected Dr. Clarence J. Gamble as its first president, from 1933 to 1936, followed by sociologist James H. S. Bossard from 1937 to 1938. In Connecticut, Episcopal minister William T. Hooper presided over its Birth Control League in 1933; all other presidents were women. When men headed these leagues the terms of office were short, unlike those of their female counterparts, who often stayed in office for decades.

African American Activists

Clinic activists were overwhelmingly white. When leagues opened clinics to serve African Americans, they often created a special advisory board of local black leaders, but rarely invited these activists to join the main board or to volunteer at the clinic. We do not know enough about the small number of African American operated clinics, but my sense is that they were organized much like white clinics, with women doing the brunt of the work and men lending their names and specific professional skills.[31]

Despite the fact that most clinics in the 1920s had no formal policies banning African American patients, the combination of location, a lack of encouragement, and the racial politics of American cities made it obvious that white activists were uncomfortable with African Americans and most were unwilling to take the steps necessary to change. Operating in a society that was largely segregated, the white women who ran clinics did not feel responsible for providing charity for African Americans. Many expected that a parallel movement, headed by a middle-class African American woman, would evolve to tend to the needs of poor black women. While African American activists engaged in a wide variety of social reforms, including anti-lynching campaigns and fights for equal rights and opportunities, they concentrated on winning the most basic reforms for the health of African American mothers and children, not on birth control. Faced with inadequate medical resources, black women's clubs worked to establish black hospitals, medical schools, and training for nurses, teachers, and social workers. African American women were not encouraged to work with white activists, who could be condescending. White activists often snubbed African Americans, whether social workers, doctors, nurses, or clergymen, by segregating them. While prominent African Americans were often willing, when invited, to help foster clinics in black neighborhoods, they behaved more like lay men, advising on and approving work done by others, but rarely volunteering their time or money. What's more, African Americans did not develop their own national or state birth control leagues to address inequity in contraceptive access. Most supported birth control, but none made it the center of their activism.[32] This led to a situation where African American women who wanted to control their family size had less information, less help, and less encouragement than their white counterparts.

Many African Americans were suspicious of white efforts to spread birth control in their neighborhoods. They associated contraception with sterilization or abortion, and distrusted some of the activists' motives. Others believed that large families were a positive thing, a measure of stature in the community and of God's blessings.[33]

Harlem provides an example of the limitations of unequal interracial cooperation. As early as 1918, the Harlem Women's Political Association offered lectures on birth control, and by 1923 Sanger was invited before the Harlem Community Forum.[34] Unlike clinics in other cities, Sanger's BCCRB accepted African American patients, though its location made it difficult for many Harlem women to use. Only 3 percent of the BCCRB's patients were black in 1929.[35] Harlem leaders wanted a clinic in their own neighborhood, run by and for African Americans. In 1929, African American social worker James H. Hubert, executive secretary of New York's Urban League, approached Sanger to discuss opening a branch clinic in Harlem. This was a second attempt at a Harlem clinic; in 1925 efforts to open a clinic in the Columbus Hill section failed due to low attendance. Unlike some other clinics created in African American neighborhoods, the Harlem Branch was not restricted to blacks; it also served white patients from the northern region of the city. Opened in February 1930 with the backing of Harlem's elite, the branch clinic had its own fifteen-member advisory board of African American doctors, clergymen, nurses, journalists, and social workers who advised and promoted the clinic.[36] The clinic was publicized in the African American press, in the pulpits of some of Harlem's most respected churches, and through medical channels. Sanger funded the clinic through grants from the Chicago-based Julius Rosenwald Fund and the donations of other white donors.[37] The Harlem Branch treated 1,737 patients in its first year, about half of them African Americans. Sanger continued funding the branch, asking its advisory council to focus on ways of increasing black attendance. The council broadened publicity efforts, replaced some white staff with African Americans, and eventually moved the clinic to the Urban League building, both to reduce expenses and to encourage community trust. In better economic times, the Harlem Branch might have prospered, but its timing was poor. The Depression made it extremely difficult to break even, as patient numbers rose with the spiraling unemployment rates. Patients could only afford to pay less for the services than previously, raising the amounts that Sanger had to provide for staff and supplies. Donations were down and charities were deluged with requests for aid. Among African Americans the situation was extremely dire, as they were often the first fired and last in line to receive government and private relief. During the 1930s, Sanger's fund-raising was stretched to operate both BCCRB clinics, as well as the NCFLBC's extensive lobbying efforts in Washington. Even in the best of times, Sanger's clinic model, with paid staff and doctors and open many hours per week, was expensive. It depended on outside funding and volunteers to break even.

Sanger sought aid from the Harlem Advisory Council as early as 1932, hoping that they would accept financial responsibility for the clinic. Comprised of doctors, lawyers, and clergymen like the BCCRB's board, what the

Harlem council lacked were wealthy philanthropists, socialites, or club women who could open their wallets to quickly cover deficits or put in hours of volunteer work at the clinic.[38] As such, the Harlem council was unwilling (or unable) to take financial responsibility. As one of the council members, nursing leader Mabel Keaton Staupers, noted, African American donors had "so many demands that the entire responsibility of operating a clinic would seem to me to be impossible."[39] The Harlem clinic limped along until 1935, when the Julius Rosenwald Fund did not renew its aid. Sanger threatened to close the clinic unless the council would help her fund it, and though they urged her not to close it, the council again refused to support it themselves. Looking for a way out, both Sanger and the council jumped when the ABCL offered to take over the clinic. In June of 1936 the clinic was renamed and reorganized with a smaller budget and less-frequent sessions, and it continued into the 1940s.[40]

It may be true that the Harlem Advisory Council could not fully fund the clinic, though based on the budgets of some other clinics either they or Sanger certainly could have reorganized it to run more cheaply. Using their connections in the Harlem community, the council could have secured volunteer doctors, nurses, and social workers to staff the clinic's reduced hours. Fund-raising at Harlem churches might have covered supply costs. But these common tactics required a commitment of time and energy from at least one individual. The Harlem clinic had to become someone's top priority, and that did not happen. The Harlem council valued birth control and thought it would benefit their community, but it was only one among a mountain of needs and not the most important.[41]

Why didn't the African American activists in Harlem and other cities value birth control clinics as highly as white activists did? African American activists were deeply concerned about the health and welfare of poor black women and their children. Both infant and maternal mortality rates among African Americans were significantly higher than those of whites because of discrimination and a lack of access to quality health care. Black patients were refused access to many charity hospitals. Black doctors and nurses could only attend a limited number of schools and could only work in segregated hospitals. Public officials often discriminated against African Americans when doling out assistance. To address these inequities, black professionals established medical schools, hospitals, and charities to provide services denied African Americans.[42] While birth control was pitched and understood as a tool to improve health, reduce mortality rates, and provide economic breathing space, it was also a loaded topic for many African Americans, who associated it with genocide, race suicide, and white control over African American fertility. Intellectuals like W. E. B. Du Bois and Mary McLeod Bethune supported efforts to extend birth control to the black community for the same reasons that white intellectuals did, but it seems that black club women found birth control easier to practice than to preach. Opposition to birth control came from black nationalist Marcus Garvey and from the pulpits of some Baptist ministers, who portrayed birth control as sinful or detrimental to the best interests of the race.[43] In many ways, mirroring Sanger's early radical claims for birth control, middle-class African Americans supported it as a means to raise living standards enough to gain the time and resources to fight larger battles for equality. Carole McCann argues that African American professionals valued birth control, but as a secondary aim, never equal to civil rights. She also argued that African American women's desire to be seen as "respectable" made it less likely that they would risk volunteering at a birth control clinic.[44]

No African American reformer took up the challenge to become a "Margaret Sanger for her people."[45] Nor did any black organization step up to redress the failings of white activists and provide clinic services for African American women. When white activists approached them, African American women's groups cooperated, lending space, securing referrals, and occasionally providing partial funding, but they rarely took the lead. Black women did not create birth control organizations at the local, state, or national level to mirror the white groups, nor did they press the white leadership to grant them equal access to existing organizations. Middle-class African American activists were concerned by birth control's associations with promiscuity and immorality. They also tended to prefer working on securing black participation in middle-class reform movements over working directly with poor African American women.[46]

Despite the inclusion of prominent African Americans on special advisory boards, birth control leagues and clinics were not interracial organizations. Prominent African Americans were not invited to join lay or medical advisory groups created for integrated or white-centered clinics, nor were they asked to join national medical committees. This is a familiar pattern, common to many social reforms, but it added yet another obstacle to African American participation. Some African American reformers complained of a lack of respect from their white counterparts, and it certainly seems that the white movement was more interested in crafting lists of prominent African Americans than it was in actually listening to them. After the ABCL took over the Harlem Branch, Mabel Keaton Staupers, head of the National Association of Colored Graduate Nurses, complained to Sanger that the ABCL leaders looked "on us as children to be cared for and not to help us decide how the caring should be done." Staupers argued that "if any work is being done for Negroes in any community, Negroes should share in the planning and in the expense to the best of their ability."[47] Six years later, Dorothy Boulding Ferebee echoed the same lament, advising white activists that "the Negro at his present advanced state of development is increasingly interested more in programs that are worked out with and by him, than in those worked out for him."[48] White activists nodded their heads at these sentiments in the 1930s, but there is little sense that they took them to heart or worked to include African Americans in planning and operating their clinics and leagues.

Though most birth control clinics were sponsored by white activists, there were a few clinics operated by and for African Americans.[49] Very little documentation on these clinics is available. Most were small in scale, located in the homes of social workers or in community centers or churches. They did not get widespread newspaper coverage, did not print brochures or reports, and had little contact with white-dominated birth control leagues at the city, state, or national level. Many were organized by only one or two individuals, without the support of a league. Yet they were out there, perhaps in greater numbers than we know. Much as would have occurred in a white neighborhood, the Baltimore Urban League gathered fifteen "key" women to form the core of a clinic committee, eventually expanding the group into a committee of one hundred "physicians, dentists, pharmacists, nurses, social workers, lawyers, teachers, journalists, housewives, business men, labor leaders, and heads of civic and fraternal organizations" to sponsor the clinic. In an article discussing their tactics, organizers E. S. Lewis and Louise Young reported, "It is important to organize clinics for colored people from the top of the leadership pyramid down,"[50] thus refuting the notion that African Americans organized in a more egalitarian, grassroots manner. In Miami, social worker Evelyn Boggs founded the Mother's Health Clinic for the Colored in her home. She persuaded a county health physician, Dr. Frederick Douglass Mazon, to refer patients to the clinic, and he also occasionally fitted women with pessaries there. Most patients, however, were treated with foam powder contraceptives by Boggs at the clinic and by another social worker, Vern Harris, who visited women in their homes. A "financial man," William Tate, tried to raise contributions to keep the clinic going.[51] In Oklahoma City, the Brockway Recreation Center Clinic offers an example of a clinic organized with help from the local birth control league. In this case, an association of fourteen African American women's clubs funded the clinic. In California, there were several clinics that were never listed in the national directories, including the Los Angeles Outdoor Life and Health Association and the Ruth J. Temple Institute. A physician, Temple directed the Los Angeles Division of Specialized Health Services and had lobbied for a public health center in southeastern Los Angeles. Rebuffed, she opened her own clinic, which offered birth control along with pre- and postnatal care. The Outdoor Life Clinic was a tuberculosis treatment center that added contraception to its services.[52] Mentions of these kinds of clinics, ephemeral and not closely linked with the national or state leagues, hint at a much broader clinic experience than can be readily documented.[53]

As more work is done to uncover the stories of individual clinics and leagues, a richer portrait of lay birth control activists emerges. But lay women were not the only ones who made birth control clinics work. Though their roles were crucial, without medical allies their work would have remained clandestine and illegal.

Medical Activists

Doctors were critical to the success of the clinic movement. Lay activists were careful to maintain cordial relations with local medical societies to secure staff and prevent opposition. Organized medicine, dominated by white men, distrusted both extramural clinics and birth control, which meant that activists had to develop policies to answer doctors' objections. Sanger, in particular, appealed to physicians, backing "doctors-only" bills to exempt the medical profession from prosecution under the Comstock Act. She opposed liberal bills that sought to legalize contraception for everyone because she did not believe that such a broad reform could win. At the local level, activists avoided conflict with local medical societies. In a "divide and conquer" strategy, they worked on one doctor at a time, winning converts to their cause and only then seeking the approval of medical societies. By the mid-1930s, with the success of lobbying and propaganda efforts, clinics sought a more formal relationship with prominent physicians, though these doctors did not actually work with clinics.

The doctors who actively supported the birth control movement did so for a variety of reasons. Most believed that birth control would directly improve the health of the women who used it. Some physicians came to the movement from backgrounds in public health, convinced that women suffering from tuberculosis and other chronic diseases were too weakened to bear children.[54] Others argued that malnutrition led to high infant and maternal mortality rates and posited that birth control could allow the poor to space children so that they were more affordable. Doctors also accepted eugenic rationales that birth control would improve the quality of the population by reducing the transmission of hereditary diseases. And many women physicians operated on the feminist belief that women knew best when and if they should have children. Unlike eugenicists and some lay activists, who looked generally to see how birth control could better society, physicians often focused on how the information would improve the lives of their individual patients.

More so than their lay counterparts, the physicians associated with birth control clinics can be divided into two groups—those who worked at the clinics and those who advised them. Despite their common profession, these two groups did not share equal status at the clinic. Women doctors were often found working at the clinics, while the vast majority of advisors were men.[55] Clinicians, the staff physicians, and medical directors of the clinics were the more varied group, comprising men and women at all stages of their careers.

Using a sampling of clinic staff lists, of 1,098 clinicians whose gender could be identified, 555, or just over 50 percent, were men (see table 2). As women made up only between 3 and 6 percent of medical school enrollees between 1905 and 1928, the position of birth control clinician was distinctly feminized.[56] Institutional clinics were more likely to employ men because they were drawing from existing staff. Almost two-thirds of clinicians at hospital and public health clinics were men, while in the female dominion

Table 2. Percentage of Clinicians by Gender and Clinic Type

Clinic Type	Women	Men
Settlement	72%	28%
Independent	52%	48%
Government	36%	64%
Hospital	35%	65%

Sources: Compiled from league letterheads, reports, brochures, and other sources.

of settlement clinics almost three-quarters of physicians were women. In most cases clinics hired only one doctor, which meant that in less-populated areas there were few women physician candidates. Woman doctors were easier to find in the industrial cities of the Northeast and Midwest and the booming California cities. Many independent clinics, such as the BCCRB and the IBCL clinics, purposefully hired all-women medical staffs. Activists, even those in the medical profession, believed that women doctors were better suited to the task. CMHA clinician Sarah Marcus admitted that even she was embarrassed when being examined by a male gynecologist, and believed that male doctors were at a disadvantage "because they can't be as intimate with [patients] as a woman can be. I can put my finger in her vagina with her finger and show her just what she's supposed to know and demonstrate it, but a man doctor doesn't do that. He's hesitant to do it, it's a little bit too aggressive for a woman to have a man do this to her. So I think it's a field that a woman physician, and only a woman physician does properly."[57]

A few clinicians became well known and respected in the birth control movement for their research work, but most were simply employees of the clinic, and as such were not invited to become league or clinic officers, members of its board, or of the medical advisory committees. Even the clinic's medical director, who held ultimate responsibility for patient care, in many cases was not a member of the medical committee that determined the clinic's procedures and policies. Gender does seem to have mattered here; male clinicians and medical directors were more likely to sit on the advisory group than women. Most female clinicians were doubly marginalized—both in terms of the power structure at the clinic and within the medical profession. The career of Hannah Mayer Stone, arguably the most experienced clinician in the country, offers a telling example. Stone began her association with the BCCRB in 1925; prior to that she had worked at a variety of New York hospitals and shared a joint practice with her husband, Abraham. Like many clinicians, she was not an obstetrician/gynecologist; instead she had trained as a bacteriologist and serologist before completing her medical degree. Stone combined her private practice with extensive volunteer work at the BCCRB and the Newark Birth Control Clinic, until her sudden death in 1941. As medical director of the busiest birth control clinic in the country, she gathered and interpreted more clinical data than anyone else. She supervised both contraceptive testing and training programs for physicians, social workers, and visitors from around the country and the world. Especially during the early 1930s, Stone ran the BCCRB. Her research was published in pamphlets, in conference proceedings, in clinic reports, in the *Journal of Contraception*, and in the occasional minor medical journal.[58]

Despite this prominence, Stone had difficulty gaining the respect of the larger medical community. As a Jewish woman associated with birth control, doctors distrusted her. They suspected that she and other clinicians simply allowed lay women the use of their professional credentials to provide promiscuous access to contraception. Stone was regularly shunned by the local medical society, lost hospital privileges because of her birth control work, and acquired what was later described as a "bad odor" with the new male physicians brought into the national movement at the end of the 1930s. As national leaders tried to forge better relations with doctors, Stone's lack of medical prestige became an excuse to limit her responsibility at the national level. Never was this more obvious than when the BCFA, formed by the merger of the BCCRB and the ABCL in 1939, created its medical committees. It was Hannah Stone's husband, urologist Abraham Stone, who was invited to join, despite his limited birth control experience. Hannah Stone was never considered for the position of BCFA medical director; instead a lengthy search was undertaken to find a male "name" to confer prestige on the organization and impress medical men.[59] When Stone died suddenly in 1941, Sanger recalled that she "was at times left out of this group—pushed off this committee—ignored when she should be recognized. Her work, discoveries, methods snapped up by others with more prominent names & used to their own advantage. Doubtless she must have been hurt, doubtless she must have felt the pangs of the knife thrust through the heart—but never did I hear her beg or ask favors for herself or criticize others for these things. Always she laughed at the reasons given & the methods behind these acts."[60]

Hannah Stone's career provides an example of the different skills valued by the national movement and by local clinics. At the BCCRB, Stone was revered, on a par with Sanger herself. As described by Sanger, she had "a sympathetic response to mothers in distress, and a broad attitude toward life's many problems. . . . These qualities have kept her with us all this time, one of the most beloved and loyal workers that one could ever hope for."[61] But Stone's expertise and her close association with Sanger over the years made her a liability to the national birth control movement, not an asset. Her close association with and understanding of the movement was not what the national birth control movement was looking for; instead they wanted respected doctors, even if they were birth control neophytes, to lend the movement credibility.

Clinicians like the IBCL's Rachelle Slobodinsky Yarros, who limited her interest to local clinics and public health medicine, did not face the same disappointments. Like Stone and several other prominent clinicians, Yarros was Jewish, and may have had very limited avenues for traditional professional positions.[62] She did not attempt to compete with medical men on their own terms, but rather kept her work specifically focused on women's activism. A Russian immigrant with a radical political background, Yarros dedicated her career to working-class women's health, a field shunned by most male physicians. Before working for birth control, she had opened an obstetrical program for ghetto women, become a resident of Hull House, and founded the American Social Hygiene Association. She sought the aid of wealthy women from the General Federation of Women's Clubs to fund better health education and legislation for the poor. With its close connection with the settlement, the IBCL tapped Yarros's expertise when it began planning its clinics. She became the medical director for its extensive network of clinics. In this woman-centered environment, Yarros's career as a birth control clinician differed from Stone's. She did not compete with male researchers by conducting contraceptive research, instead working to expand clinical services to as many Chicago women as possible. Her articles on birth control did not deal with clinical data or contraceptive testing; instead she made political and social arguments for birth control, based on her status as a physician. She did not seek power in the national movement, but she was respected within the IBCL. She was not only the medical director, but was also a member of the all-woman medical committee, and the IBCL Board of Directors. By treating her clinical work as an extension of her medical practice and political beliefs, Yarros found a rewarding career as a clinician and local activist.[63]

Sarah Marcus, a gynecologist at the CMHA, found that her gender blocked advancement. She started a private practice in an immigrant Polish neighborhood where they "seem to know that a woman doctor has a place in medicine." Before she joined the CMHA, Marcus partnered with a male doctor who prescribed stem pessaries (an early intrauterine device); but neither of them had any experience with diaphragms. At Cleveland's Mount Sinai Hospital, Marcus felt ostracized: "On the whole, male doctors didn't give me a helping hand. They did anything but." Marcus claimed that the doctors pushed her around, "not giving me the opportunity, criticizing me for things that weren't true, calling me an abortionist when being an abortionist was horrible . . . connected with that terrible Planned Parenthood, which Mt.

Sinai had nothing to do with, wouldn't consider at all." Marcus left Mount Sinai for a place that hired women doctors, the Woman's Hospital, founded to treat the poor. There she was finally able to advance; she became chief of the obstetrics and gynecology department and eventually vice president and later hospital president.[64] Her colleague at the CMHA, Ruth Robishaw Rauschkolb, had a similar story. Trained in dermatology, she could not secure a hospital appointment and worked in private practice with her husband until his death. Then she patched together positions at the CMHA and a public health clinic.[65]

Birth control clinics offered a rare place where women doctors were more desirable. As Dr. Thomas Parke, the medical supervisor for New York City's settlement house clinics, acknowledged, "Often our physician is the only one the patients have seen in many years. Women clinicians are used entirely because the patients are used to midwives and are afraid of men doctors."[66] Faced with difficulties securing full-time work in hospitals, many women doctors took on a variety of part-time jobs to get by. Birth control clinics offered a viable option for some, though the pay was often low. Many clinicians were not trained in obstetrics and gynecology, but were refugees from discrimination in a wide variety of medical specialties.

For some clinicians birth control became an integral part of their professional lives. The names of the same women pepper the staff lists for a number of different clinics. Doctors such as Nadina Reinstein Kavinoky, a trained gynecologist, supervised fifteen Los Angeles County Public Health clinics and the Pasadena Woman's Hospital clinic. In New York, Doctor Elizabeth Pissoort, a Belgian-born gynecologist, was one of the physicians arrested when the BCCRB was raided in 1929.[67] Pissoort was all the more unique because she was able to remain above the intense rivalry between Sanger and the ABCL, working for clinics sponsored by both.

Despite the fact that patients preferred women doctors, clinics could not always hire them. In Little Rock there were 235 male physicians, but only 7 women physicians practiced. Because they feared losing what little status they had, few women doctors were willing to work at the clinic.[68] At the BCCRB, Sanger's insistence on women doctors meant that in the early years candidates were not always well qualified. Willingness and enthusiasm were often easier to secure than obstetrical or gynecological credentials.[69]

But male clinicians were not marginalized like women were. Better off financially, they had traditional medical respectability—hospital appointments, memberships in medical societies, and successful private practices.

While some complained that their association with birth control cost them patients, particularly among Roman Catholics, it was less likely to jeopardize their professional affiliations.[70] It seems that the community of doctors looked upon a male doctor at a birth control clinic as a brake upon the sentimentality of lay women activists, while women doctors were assumed to be selling their professional brethren out, either for money or for feminist ideas.

In the few instances where women served both as officers and clinicians, they were usually the founder of the clinic, such as the cases of Dr. Adelaide Brown at the San Francisco Educational Center and Lydia Allen deVilbiss at the Miami Mother's Health Clinics. A handful of male clinicians became leaders in birth control leagues. Dr. Abraham Nowell Creadick, an obstetrician and gynecologist on the faculty at Yale University, served as president and vice president of the Connecticut Birth Control League while also contributing time on staff. Robert J. Crossen, an obstetrician and gynecologist on the staff of eight different local hospitals as well as the faculty of Washington University's Medical School, did the same for the St. Louis Maternal Health League. At the Indianapolis Maternal Health Clinic, Charles Owen McCormick served on both the board of directors, the clinic committee, and as medical director. A Harvard-trained obstetrician, he was on the faculty of the Indiana University Medical School, with privileges in a number of local hospitals. Though McCormick did not treat clinic patients, he and the other committee members hired and supervised the male clinician and authored the clinic's annual reports, published in the *Indiana State Medical Journal.* When he stepped down after two years, clinician Austin S. Johnson became medical director, and was also invited to join the board of directors, receiving the kind of deference from the lay women who ran the clinic that a female clinician like Hannah Stone never did. Throughout his association with the clinic, Johnson maintained his existing professional affiliations and suffered no obvious professional setback for his association with birth control.[71]

Young male clinicians sometimes used birth control work to help establish themselves in private practice. In Connecticut, the two male clinicians at the Waterbury Hospital Maternal Health Clinic were newly minted obstetricians who had only recently moved to Hartford. William Goodrich was pressed into service by Clara McTernan, the executive secretary of the birth control league. He had worked in a birth control clinic while in medical school and may have seen the clinic as a way to build a Waterbury-based medical practice. Another recent graduate, Roger Nelson, was also looking to set up a practice. For these young doctors, volunteering at a birth control clinic provided experience and connections they hoped would advance their careers.[72] Clarence Gamble believed that while hiring women doctors was preferable, if a clinic could not obtain one it should go after "young and ambitious males."[73]

Male clinicians were especially influential at hospital clinics, most of which had no formal lay or medical committee to supervise their work. These services often began when a staff doctor grafted birth control services onto an existing outpatient department. At Mount Sinai Hospital in New York, the key player was gynecology chief Dr. Max Mayer, who agreed to cooperate with the CMH as early as 1925. Mount Sinai's service never had official recognition, produced little literature or studies, and was characterized within the hospital as Mayer's hobby.[74] Doctors at hospital clinics had little contact with the birth control movement or other clinicians, they did not attend the conferences, and it is unlikely that their participation in institutional clinics much affected their advancement at their institutions.

Most male doctors held advisory positions at clinics. Of 324 members of medical advisory boards in a sampling of clinics, 265, or 82 percent, were male, not surprising given the goal of the boards—to cooperate and consult with established doctors in each city.[75] Securing such support helped blunt organized medical opposition that might threaten a clinic. Very few of these physicians took an active role in leagues.[76]

At the local medical society, male clinic advisors received a more cordial welcome than women doctors did. When St. Louis Medical Society members objected to a circular letter seeking information about physicians willing to accept birth control patients, Dr. Robert Crossen stepped up to explain things to the society.[77] In Youngstown, Ohio, despite the creation of a seven-member medical advisory board, the County Medical Society opposed the clinic and threatened to oust any member who associated with it. The clinic closed for three months in 1928 while its medical board lobbied members of the society. When reconstituted, the clinic had gained more than the sufferance of the society, it had their blessing. Rather than have a few volunteer doctors staff the clinic, the society organized a larger panel of doctors to volunteer time on a rotating basis. The new relationship was so successful that the clinic had to add new sessions because of the unexpected numbers of patients referred from the Medical Society.[78] It is unlikely that this kind of reaction would have resulted had the advisory committee been composed of women physicians. When Hannah Stone sought admission to the New York County Medical Society, she found the members hostile and prejudiced, describing an adversarial interview "so much like one of those hearings in Albany or Washington." Asked about her policy of admitting women to the clinic on medical grounds for child spacing, she noted "a definite note of disapproval" and was closely questioned on the medical authorities that she based her decisions on.[79]

Lay and Medical Relations

The lay women who founded birth control clinics faced a dilemma. While many seasoned activists contended that birth control was a woman's issue and responsibility, all acknowledged that to be effective, it needed support from men. Never was this more obvious than in the 1930s, when efforts to amend the Comstock Laws and include birth control in public health programs foundered on a lack of access to traditional political power. It is in this context that birth control activists stepped up campaigns to secure the support of physicians, clergymen, and politicians, even though it meant ceding some control over the movement.

But most lay activists viewed the clinics as their preserve and did not necessarily let medical personnel dictate how care would be offered. As Margaret Sanger opined in 1932, "The doctors consider that what they do to the patient is none of anyone's particular business; that they should have carte blanche to 'treat the patient as they wish.' I assure you the doctor who holds that attitude very long does not stay in the Clinical Research Bureau while MS is Director."[80]

Sanger was more likely able to enforce such a policy than other activists, but her attitude was not unique. Lay activists saw birth control as a cause. When a physician joined the clinic's staff, whether as a volunteer or paid employee, he or she was expected to adopt the cause and adhere to the clinic's policies. Physicians who did not meet these standards were replaced. BCCRB clinician Sarah Kelman once refused to treat a patient, most likely for a lack of medical cause, and was fired. Sanger defended her decision by writing Hannah Stone: "I would never rest one day away from the clinic to have a doctor like this dictating terms to any of the patients. I do not think a reprimand is sufficient—only a dismissal will set the standard straight for such a serious error as this is."[81]

Directives from both the ABCL and the BCCRB encouraged clinics to secure more participation from male doctors, businessmen, and government officials.[82] In order to secure such support, they recast their organizations in terms that men would respect. In their effort to "professionalize," the ABCL in particular denigrated the value of lay women's participation at clinics, pushing male-run hospital and public health clinics and shutting women out of all but fund-raising duties.[83] The new model, so similar to that proposed by the New York Academy of Medicine almost twenty years earlier, once again failed to take into account what patients wanted (female clinicians) and what was feasible.[84] Nor did it acknowledge that the independent clinic was the most numerous and popular clinic form precisely because it was a woman-friendly place. The press to include men in the movement shifted rhetoric toward community needs for birth control, population issues, reductions in the numbers of welfare recipients, and infertility research. Lay women thought that men would be interested in fostering "better babies," rather than fewer babies, and did not want to pitch contraceptives as offering liberating freedoms for women. CMHA Executive Secretary Gladys Gaylord delineated two paths in a speech to the Pennsylvania Birth Control Federation in 1939, claiming that one way to go was the route taken by Sanger, to make birth control a cause and life's goal and risk everything for that. Noting that few were capable of that kind of sacrifice, she outlined another route, that of marketing birth control much as you would any new idea, identifying what people care about, and positioning your movement to attract the broadest, if not the most fervent, support possible. She argued that men liked to hear calls for more children if "the physical and mental background is sound. It means fewer babies when such indications of a good heritage are not present." She characterized men as interested in the economic aspects of unwanted children, such as the costs of institutionalizing the unfit, and the increased productivity of happier workers who were not burdened by large families and ill health.[85] To Gaylord, the national leadership, and many other activists who lacked the pioneer's fire in the belly, this second approach would prove comfortable.

By the late 1930s, the national movement was changing. Especially at the ABCL, which was heavily influenced by a small group of male physicians and public relations experts, men replaced women in most offices. From its founding in 1921 to 1936, the ABCL had only three presidents: Margaret Sanger, Eleanor Dwight Jones,[86] and Catherine Clement Bangs.[87] Genetics professor Clarence Cook Little became the first male president in 1936. Under his tenure the ABCL merged with Sanger's organizations, forming the Birth Control Federation of America.[88] With the reorganization came an influx of men and the demotion of longtime women activists. The sixty-year-old Sanger was named "Honorary President," a position carrying no institutional power, while Dr. Richard Norris Pierson, an obstetrician and gynecologist, was named president pro-tem.[89] The position of real power, director, was filled in 1940 by Dr. Woodbridge E. Morris, a physician with extensive public health experience but no background in birth control.[90] Of the seven major BCFA officers in 1939, only one, the secretary, was a woman (Marguerite Benson).[91]

What happened to all the women? Most retreated willingly, seeing men's increased participation as a sign that the movement had achieved mainstream success. Women activists, Sanger included, believed that men were more effective managers, fund-raisers, and leaders and expected them to make better progress integrating clinics with medicine and public health. But in promoting men over women with experience and knowledge of the movement, the BCFA weakened its link with local activists, especially as many longtime women workers resigned from the federation within a few years.[92] Sanger, after a brief period of optimism, criticized the new leadership as tentative, finding fault with their fears of generating controversy. The board of directors, still composed of women, continued to raise funds for the BCFA, but was increasingly left out of policy decisions about how the money should be spent.

Efforts were clearly made at the national level to encourage and even mandate increased participation from male doctors at the local level, but lay women resisted the wholesale transfer of power. Rather than reject national guidelines, clinics met them without really changing their makeup. Lay women continued to open independent clinics throughout the 1930s, though they often paid lip service to the desire to have the clinic housed in an institutional setting.[93] And they did not cede control of their local birth control groups to men. Of the presidents of the twenty-eight state and local birth control leagues affiliated to the ABCL at the time of the merger in 1939, twenty-six were women. Only one was a physician (a man).[94] At the local level, national guidelines and instructions did not change the clinic's operation in any real way, though the letterhead might be weighted with a bevy of new names on fancy advisory committees.

An example is the Arkansas Eugenics Association, which over the 1930s expanded and reorganized its boards and committees, adding more men. But the officers, and the power at the clinic, remained resolutely female. In 1931, when the association was founded, the board of governors, a loose list of sponsors who never met, consisted of twenty-two prominent individuals—twelve men and ten women. As one of the avowed purposes of the board was to forge links between the clinic and the medical profession, six of the governors were physicians. Also, while it was explicitly stated that the governors had no official responsibilities, most of the female governors also served as clinic assistants. None of the male governors held any other office at the clinic. In 1934, in response to advice from the ABCL and the BCCRB, the association created a Medical Advisory Council, moving most of the physicians from the Governing Board to the new council and recruiting new members to fill out both. Three years later the Board of Governors was renamed the Board of Directors and the two groups were further divided along gender lines. Clinic work involving medicine became exclusively a male preserve overseen by the Medical Advisory Council and the clinic's medical staff. Women handled administration, daily operations, publicity, and fund-raising. They also held all offices save that of treasurer. The men met rarely and generally approved the clinic's policies, which had been set up earlier. In essence, they provided the official medical backing that the national movement required, but in practice they were neither engaged with nor involved in the clinic's work.[95]

The Arkansas example is a common one for clinics founded in the 1930s, with both men and women serving on advisory boards. But there were a significant number of older clinics that relied almost exclusively on women, both working in the clinics and on their boards. Though the IBCL was initially organized by a coalition of men and women, shortly after it opened its first clinic it became a preserve of lay women. By the late 1920s, the board of directors, officers and medical staff, and medical advisors consisted solely of women.[96] Men were permitted to join the League's Council, a publicity vehicle that neither met nor had any official duties. As silent supporters, two-thirds of the council was male, drawn mostly from the clergy and medical profession.[97]

How much of this trend came from male lack of interest? It is impossible to be sure, but it appears that men were more interested in the national level policy work, possibly because of its remove from patient care. It comes down again to the goals of the local movement, which focused less on propaganda and attracting public support, and more on treating patients. Lay and medical men could not easily step into the roles held by the lay women activists because such work was seen as inappropriate for men. While medical men were willing to advise the clinic's activists, few were so convinced of its importance that they were willing to take time away from lucrative private practices to treat charity patients. None were willing to man the admission and supply desks or visit patients in their homes. And the patients probably would not have wanted them there.

The doctors who took control of the national movement, particularly at the ABCL, showed a bullish tendency to force their own ideas about clinics without taking into account the needs and desires of the patients. They insisted on moving clinics to government health programs and hospitals, where their acceptance was lukewarm at best, creating a program that did not serve patients as well as the independent woman-controlled clinics did. In order to replace female clinic leadership, volunteer labor had to be replaced by paid workers. This increased overhead costs. Someone would have to do the jobs the volunteers had done, make the difficult choices about whether to admit women who might not meet all the admission criteria set by its medical board, or determine how much a patient might be able to afford for her care. Lay volunteer women, steeped in charity experience, felt more comfortable with such decisions, while paid employees tended to fall back on written rules without any exceptions.

Birth control began as a woman's reform movement, but clinic work demanded the participation and cooperation of the medical profession. This created tensions, both at the national level and in the operation of local clinics. The bulk of the work of organizing, funding, and staffing clinics fell to lay women, whose investments of time and money were built on a personal commitment to birth control reform. In contrast, most of the physicians who worked at the clinics did so in either a paid capacity or as advisors, and they were less committed to seeing the clinic prosper. Despite the prestige that prominent medical advisors brought their clinics, the lay women who funded and worked at the clinics controlled their destinies throughout the 1930s. This was especially true for independent clinics, where success was determined more by the ability to raise money and enthusiasm than by the support or opposition of the medical profession. Lay women at clinics ignored the national movement's efforts to replace them with doctors and professionals. They retained the clinic model that had succeeded in the past, one that relied on their labors and unique abilities and contributions.

FOUR

Eugenics and Race at the Clinic

Birth control clinics were founded during a period in American history when nativism and racism were widely accepted both by the general public and political, social, and economic leaders. The most acceptable outlet for these views was the "science" of eugenics. Birth control activists worked alongside scientists, social workers, teachers, and physicians, all of whom believed that people could be divided into categories of "fit" and "unfit" based upon their racial or ethnic backgrounds; that characteristics like "thrift" or "shiftlessness" could be inherited; and that society had a responsibility to protect its "quality" by both encouraging and discouraging growth in certain population segments.[1] Eugenicists argued that economic and intellectual successes were not the products of environmental advantage, but rather of a Darwinian survival of the fittest in a contest between those of superior and inferior heredity. Eugenics was a conservative ideology, blind to its own cultural and racial biases, that was touted as a "pure" science. In reality, its theories supported the status quo of white Anglo-Saxon supremacy against what was depicted as a "rising tide of color." Pushing a dual program of increasing the numbers of the "fit" and eliminating the "unfit," eugenicists were extremely influential in areas of immigration, education, marriage licensing, and sterilization.[2] And so, the birth control movement, especially at the national level, adopted eugenic rhetoric to gain widespread support.

It is important to understand that eugenics and eugenicists were not monolithic. Beneath the rubric "eugenicist" were a wide variety of beliefs. Labeling a birth control activist or scientist a "eugenicist" does not provide *all* the information needed to understand their views. As the debates on nature versus nurture in the 1920s showed, eugenicists pursued varied courses. Some, like Henry Fairfield Osborn and Charles Davenport, adopted a "mainline" approach that privileged heredity over all other factors. Others, such as Herbert Spencer Jennings, developed a reformist position that allowed for the importance of both environment and heredity.[3] Many well-known eugenicists held explicitly racist beliefs. Madison Grant, Lothrop Stoddard, and others at the Galton Institute promoted Nordic and Alpine peoples at the expense of Mediterraneans, Slavs, and nonwhites.[4] Others, like W. E. B. Du Bois and his "talented tenth," rejected arguments about the inherent superiority of one racial or ethnic group, but encouraged "fitness" within every community.[5] Not surprisingly, eugenicists were divided over the issue of birth control clinics. Some saw clinics as valuable tools to reduce the numbers of the "unfit," but the majority thought birth control was "dysgenic"; that the easy availability of contraceptives would lead the "fit" to reduce their numbers and would lower the "quality" of the population.[6]

The birth control and eugenics movements, though related, certainly were not seen as interchangeable in the 1920s and 1930s. Birth control was far more controversial and questionable a movement, backed by relatively unknown lay women with few political connections. Eugenics, on the other hand, was fostered by white male academics from prestigious universities, supported by philanthropists, who influenced law and education. Widely respected national leaders such as Theodore Roosevelt and Alexander Graham Bell were eugenicists. It was associated with science, reason, and dispassion, while birth control conjured up images of feminism, immorality, and emotionalism. Birth control activists, consequently, thought that eugenics could bring prestige and validation to their movement, much in the same way that they sought out the support of doctors and social workers. Draping birth control in eugenic robes made it more respectable. Activists in Little Rock purposefully named themselves the Arkansas Eugenics Association, as a less controversial choice than "Birth Control Association."[7]

Birth control's niche in the eugenics movement was in "negative eugenics," or efforts to reduce the numbers of the "unfit." Clinic flyers, reports, newspaper articles, and the speeches and testimonies of activists, all extolled birth control as an important tool in reducing the fertility of the "feebleminded," who were identified as criminals, paupers, and other drains on society. Birth control would enable the government to reduce its crippling economic burden by reducing the numbers on relief rolls and housed in state-run institutions. Many birth control activists supported other negative eugenics issues, such as immigration restriction, sterilization programs, and medical screenings for marriage licenses. Some, no doubt, agreed with racist eugenicists who denigrated the "new immigrants" and nonwhites as simply inferior.[8]

But the picture is not that simple. The practices at birth control clinics challenged basic hereditarian eugenic theory. Birth control clinics were organized around the concept that "fitness" was as much an environmental circumstance as it was a product of heredity. By simply reducing the size of a family, real improvements in lifestyle and "quality" could result, no matter who the parents were. Only a tiny percentage of patients had actual measurable hereditary diseases or disabilities; the vast majority of them were declared "unfit" only because they were poor or unwell. Operating on a patient-by-patient basis, clinics focused on the patient's needs and desires. Clinics did not, as many eugenic programs did, put the community's needs first. And birth control clinics were voluntary. The patient had to acquiesce to the treatment in order for it to be effective. Activists did control who they admitted, but only in the sense that they refused some women admission; they had no power to compel a woman to use the clinic, nor could they force anyone to use a diaphragm. Eugenic beliefs about race, ethnic groups, or measured intelligence may have been used to encourage social workers or physicians to refer certain types of patients, but it was the patient who decided to use the clinic. Though they buried most feminist arguments for birth control under layers of medical and social prose, activists held firm to the belief that their patients were best placed to decide when to have children.

Eugenics in Theory

Were birth control activists eugenicists? Or did they merely adopt eugenic theory and rhetoric to secure influential support and public approbation? While some activists fit neatly into one group or the other, the majority fall in the gray areas in between. Like most members of their social class and upbringing, activists believed that middle- and upper-class white Anglo-Saxons were superior. They saw immigrants and nonwhites en masse as less "fit," and believed that biological reasons explained the failure of these groups to succeed in the modern world. They acknowledged that there were many other reasons barring the poor from escaping their economic circumstances—a lack of education, the inability to speak English, and unequal opportunities were some—but inherited flaws were certainly not discounted. With a long tradition of charitable work and social service behind them, the women who founded birth control clinics had years of experience working with the poor. Through settlement work, Americanization programs, the social hygiene movement, charity, and public health work, these wealthy progressives tried to better the lives of the poor by offering education, health services, pure milk, and housing reform. All of these activities were aimed to improve the environment of the poor, and tempered the hereditarian view that the poor and the immigrant were a lower form of humanity.[9]

Birth control activists used hereditarian eugenic theories to offer rationales and justifications for birth control on a grand scale. In congressional testimony, speeches, annual reports, and monographs discussing the "unfit," activists proposed birth control as the answer to the critical problem of heredity. While environment was mentioned, it was downplayed because it raised controversial questions about economic reform. During testimony for a 1934 congressional bill, for example, supporters focused their arguments on the need to reduce the number of the "unfit" through contraception, claiming that it would benefit maternal and infant health and reduce government spending. The Catholic opposition challenged the notion that heredity affected the population's quality, arguing that providing fair wages would be a far more effective solution than birth control.[10]

To explain the many differences in the views of eugenicists and birth control activists, some theorize that activists used hereditarian eugenics instrumentally—that is, simply to secure support, without necessarily believing in it.[11] Others make no real distinction between birth control and eugenics, ignoring the many issues of contention between them.[12] Activists did use eugenic rhetoric; some among them supported hereditarian eugenics as well. But if the activist was truly committed to the hereditarian eugenics creed, why didn't the clinics base their work on such beliefs? If activists only mouthed eugenic homilies to secure support, why is there no sign of this duplicity in their other writings? In fact, it seems clear that activists were confused by eugenics and it is very difficult to determine what their "true" feelings on the subject might have been, especially given how eugenics has been demonized in recent years. There are no confidential surveys of activists to reveal what they actually felt about the poor, about immigrants, or about ethnic and racial minorities. All we have to go on is what they said and what they did. Sanger's example here is instructive. Her eugenic rhetoric was all over the map—though always tightly linked to birth control. In her 1914 *Family Limitation* pamphlet, she argued that the poor should use birth control as a weapon against the capitalists who would exploit their labor.[13] She never mentioned anything about "fitness" and certainly did not side with the right of the government to control the fertility of the poor. In 1919, after her European trip and meetings with Havelock Ellis and the Drysdales, she wrote:

> While I personally believe in the sterilization of the feeble-minded, the insane and syphilitic, I have not been able to discover that these measures are more than superficial deterrents when applied to the constantly growing stream of the unfit. They are excellent means of meeting a certain phase of the situation, but . . . they do not go to the bottom of the matter. Neither the mating of healthy couples nor the sterilization of certain recognized types of the unfit touches the great problem of unlimited reproduction of those whose housing, clothing, and food are all inadequate to physical and mental health. These measures do not touch those great masses, who through economic pressure populate the slums and there produce in their helplessness other helpless, diseased and incompetent masses, who overwhelm all that eugenics can do among those whose economic condition is better.[14]

At this point, Sanger still found economics the root of "fitness," but began to accept that there were hereditary concerns. In 1920, she acknowledged that foreigners had brought with them "ignorance of hygiene and modern ways of living," but described their "cell plasms" as "freighted with the potentialities of the best in Old World civilization."[15] In her 1923 testimony in the New York State Assembly, Sanger adopted a harsher tone, reporting Harry Laughlin's contentions that the "feebleminded" were numerous, reproducing at a rapid rate, and that Italians and Jews were "filling the insane asylums . . . the hospitals . . . and our feeble-minded institutions."[16] While this reference to specific ethnic groups was rare, Sanger's emphasis on the growing menace of the "feebleminded" and "unfit" continued into the 1930s. She argued that the government had a responsibility to do something to control this population explosion, suggesting that they offer birth control to those who wanted it, and for those who could or would not use contraceptives, a choice of sterilization or physical segregation. Sanger believed sterilization was superior because it did not interfere with one's sexuality or personal freedom.[17]

The key question one must ask in reading these statements is who exactly was Sanger talking about when she talked about the "feebleminded," the "degenerate," and the "unfit?" Was she talking generally about racial and ethnic groups, or about anyone too poor to afford another child? Or was she talking about a rather small group of people with hereditary defects? It simply is not clear. When specifically questioned about the German sterilization programs in 1934, she wrote: "I admire the courage of a government that takes a stand on sterilization of the unfit and second, my admiration is subject to the interpretation of the word 'unfit.' If by 'unfit' is meant the physical or mental defects of a human being, that is an admirable gesture, but if 'unfit' refers to races or religions, then that is another matter which I frankly deplore."[18]

In her critiques of eugenics, Sanger was also clear that she considered environmental causes to be more important than inherited characteristics. In *Pivot of Civilization* (1922), she complained that some eugenicists, "affirm that heredity is everything and environment nothing, yet forget that it is precisely those whose who are most universally subject to bad environment who procreate most copiously, most recklessly and most disastrously." She continued, admitting that while heredity was important, it was "fatal to elevate it to the position of an absolute."[19]

Many eugenicists and birth control activists disagreed on "positive eugenics," or efforts to encourage increased births among those considered to be "fit." While Sanger opposed such ideas, activists like ABCL president Eleanor Dwight Jones supported them, eschewing anything that might be labeled as "anti-baby." Most activists left no record of their feelings. Many were afraid to criticize publicly these ideas for fear of being labeled "dysgenic." Thus, they argued that using birth control to space the births of children might actually *increase* population figures, because those born would have a better chance to survive. Hereditarian eugenicists disagreed, arguing strenuously that when birth control was introduced into a slum area it was adopted by the more responsible members of the community. As birth control activist and eugenicist William Hazlett Upson put it bluntly in 1936, "The stupider classes of people have not learned how to prevent conception. And the stupider people have been having more children than the intelligent. This means that each generation has an average intelligence lower than the one preceding. If this keeps on, the human race will finally go back to living in trees like monkeys."[20] Eugenic birth control activists like Upson called for a two-prong program of encouraging the poor to have smaller families and promoting larger families from the educated middle class. The United States had no mothers' pensions or baby bonuses like those used in Europe to encourage fertility, leaving American eugenicists to simply exhort middle-class white women to avoid race suicide.[21] Sanger argued that this was against the natural inclinations of parents, complaining that eugenicists "fail to recognize that this restraint of fecundity is due to a deliberate foresight and is a conscious effort to elevate the standards of living for the family and the children of the responsible—and possibly more selfish—sections of the community. The appeal to enter again into competitive child-bearing, for the benefit of the nation, or the race, or any other abstraction, will fall on deaf ears."[22]

At the birth control clinic there were no positive eugenics programs. Clinics did not try to dissuade healthy women from seeking contraceptives or promote increased fertility for those in the middle class. Indeed, until research on artificial insemination became more common in the 1940s, clinics did not address the question of infertility either. I have found only one instance in which a birth control activist, Dr. Robert Latou Dickinson, refused advice to a patient based on a eugenic evaluation that she was of "good stock" and ought to be *having* children, not delaying them.[23]

Birth control's feminist roots also put it at odds with some of the tenets of eugenics. Activists believed that the woman was the best arbiter of need, a rationale that went against eugenicists' reliance on expert evaluations. Immigration restriction, for example, relied on the idea that certain racial or ethnic groups were inherently less "fit" than others. In practice, immigration authorities employed official inspectors to identify, by observation only, "feebleminded," diseased, or otherwise undesirable aliens. Sterilization programs, especially those in state hospitals or prisons, also relied on such evaluations to identify patients "unfit" to reproduce. These evaluations were often tainted by race, class, or moral biases and rarely introduced any objective or measurable scientific tests. The best-known case was that of Carrie Buck, whose poverty, perceived promiscuity, and family history labeled her a "feebleminded" danger to society who had to be sterilized.[24]

Eugenicists believed that determinations of fitness should be made by experts, certainly not by the "unfit" themselves, especially if they were women. Eugenicists often characterized middle-class and educated women as selfish, while lower-income women were seen as feckless. They feared that if any intelligent woman had her choice, she would choose fewer children. As one irate husband and father of six ranted, "I was well able to give my children every advantage. My wife had everything any woman could ask for. But pregnancy and the care of babies interfered with her social affairs such as dinners and Bridge etc."[25] Working-class women, eugenicists contended, had little interest in contraception because they lacked forethought and were of low moral character. While birth control clinic activists shared the concern that they were not reaching the very "bottom of the barrel," they did not seek to make birth control compulsory. They did not go into slums to pressure women directly. Instead, they limited their efforts to reaching out to the "unfit" through their connections with social workers and hospitals.[26]

Practical Eugenics

Hereditarian eugenics may have been preached, but it wasn't practiced at birth control clinics. For all the talk about the menace of the "unfit," when clinic activists came face- to-face with patients they treated them as individuals—not as representatives of groups that threatened the quality of humanity. Talking with and counseling poor women complicated simple hereditarian assumptions and demonstrated that even one environmental change—ceasing unwanted pregnancies—could make a dramatic difference in a woman's life. As a clinic nurse reported, twenty-nine-year-old Mary Flores "was going crazy, with a child every year—becoming pregnant a year and one month following the birth of each child. She was small and frail and timid and apprehensive." But after attending the Tucson birth control clinic, she "is now enjoying married life without the constant fear of pregnancy. She is happy and has gained in flesh and bright in spirit."[27] This kind of casework sorely tested the faith that "fitness" came solely from bad genes. Instead, daily confrontations with the impact of poverty on women's health drove activists toward an environmental solution.

Comparing voluntary contraception and sterilization helps clarify differences in attitudes. Both procedures stopped the "unfit" from having children—sterilization permanently and birth control temporarily. Most birth control activists believed, as Sanger did in 1932, that "there are certain men and women to whom sterilization should be promptly applied—especially under those conditions where a transmissible disease or a marked mental deficiency or where the mentality is so low that the simple instruction of birth control can not be carried out." But, she continued, "I do not think sterilization can solve the whole problem alone. There are millions of normal women who desire to practice birth control, not only as a health expedient but for economic reasons as well. . . . It would not be wise to apply sterilization for such reasons."[28] Activists thought their patients could become "fit" once their economic situation was improved. They argued for child spacing, not that patients should never have another child. They argued that after a few years of childlessness a family might want another child because economic prospects had improved. Even though activists used hereditarian eugenics when discussing long-term policy and the abstract benefits of contraception, when it concerned their clinics what they offered patients was some control over their environment.[29]

Activists were less eager than eugenicists to claim that they could discern fitness. My sense is that one could support eugenic ideals in the abstract—without necessarily putting them into practice in casework. Discussions about the "unfit" were abstract; each individual interpreted the category as strictly or loosely as they chose. At the clinic, trying to measure fitness took a back seat. As Sanger commented in 1922, "We should here recognize the difficulties presented by the idea of 'fit' and 'unfit.' Who is to decide this question? The grosser, the more obvious, the undeniably feeble-minded should, indeed, not only be discouraged but prevented from propagating their kind. But among the writings of the representative Eugenists one cannot ignore the distinct middle-class bias that prevails."[30]

Sanger was not alone in criticizing the objectivity of eugenic measures of fitness, especially when applied to racial or ethnic groups. In most clinics, activists avoided making these difficult determinations by requiring their patients to come to the clinic on their own or by asking for references—in essence foisting the responsibility on social workers, doctors, or clergymen.[31] They rarely sought out the "unfit." In 1930, Caroline Robinson outlined two tactics that some clinics tried. In Denver and Los Angeles, activists worked closely with existing charities and hospitals to funnel the "unfit" to the clinic. Robinson preferred this method over tactics used by clinics in New York and Chicago. There, aggressive publicity campaigns drew in large numbers of patients, attracting more of the "fit" and the "unfit" alike.[32] In both types of clinics, most patients were there because of economic or health reasons, not social or eugenic criteria. And most patients were not referred to clinics by experts; instead they were most commonly referred by other patients, in numbers easily outdistancing referrals by social workers and medical professionals.[33]

This is not to say that activists did not use the language of eugenics to describe their patients; they most certainly did. Case reports are peppered with terms like "feebleminded," "of low mental and moral level," or "mentally defective." The public agreed to restrict the fertility of those whose children suffered from birth defects, whose husbands were criminals or alcoholics, or who were themselves either physically, mentally, or morally abnormal. In some instances, such cases were extremely compelling, as in Tucson, where: "One has only to look at the two pictures of this tragic family and see the misery they face daily. No words of mine can describe the poignancy of the condition of Raymond, age 3 who was born with seven fingers on each hand. . . . Of his poor little stumps of feet—from what would be the knee there is just a small portion and then the ankle starts but the feet which resemble a frogs are turned inward. He can creep and tries to stand on the poor little stumps. Young as he is and poor as they are he has a pride and is ashamed of his deformity, realizing too early the tragic part he is now playing in life."[34] In another instance, a woman wrote to Sanger seeking contraceptive advice: "I will be thirty-six years old on December 16, 1932, and I shall have been married fifteen years. . . . During this time I have given birth to eleven children, of whom four are now living—a boy of 13½ years—a girl of 12 years and twin boys two years old. Three of these eleven children were born badly deformed—one with a hare lip and split palate and two with excessive water and a frog-like form. The last birth (one of the deformed ones) was in August 1931 and had to be accomplished with instruments and the Doctor (E. H. Judd) feared for my life and warned us against further pregnancy. We are now living in a state of perpetual fear and anxiety and if you can aid us in preventing further conception, we will be everlastingly grateful."[35]

Other clinics reported on patients with histories of insanity, "feeblemindedness," hereditary disorders, debilitating diseases, prior histories of abortion, mentally retarded children, malnourishment, or wild and uncontrollable children.[36] In South Carolina, the State Public Health Department studied maternal mortality and concluded that 25 percent of the women who died in childbirth were "chronically unfit for the hazards of pregnancy." The study blamed repeated pregnancies, combined with poor diet and health care, for the increased risk of death.[37] Activists played up these cases, though they averaged only 10 percent of all cases.[38]

A few clinics were more explicit in measuring fitness than others. In Miami, the Mothers' Health Clinic's health visitors used eugenic categories to describe patients as either "in good physical and mental health" or "feeble-minded, diseased and psychopathic." Miami's director, Lydia deVilbiss, advised sterilization for the latter group and birth control for the former.[39] At others, birth controllers rejected the notion that they could determine who was eugenically fit. In 1934, Rachelle Yarros quipped that she didn't know who the privileged were and guessed that in five years they might not be the same people.[40] Most clinics fell between these two extremes. Clinic workers could be critical of their patients' efforts to keep their homes clean, might joke about their religious beliefs and practices, and could doubt that some patients were capable of using a complex method such as the diaphragm. Tucson clinic worker Mary Hughston, for example, blithely evaluated the home of an African American patient, as "rather above average and the children are neat and clean—a piano, a radio, happiness. She is very happy and the children bright and eager. Great contrast to the weepy pitifully weak little Mexicans and the filth and dirt of the average poor Mexican home."[41] Demonstrating an ignorance of the lives of poor people, clinic workers often found it easy to fall back on ill-defined terms like "feebleminded" or "unfit" when faced with cultural practices or values alien to their own. A BCCRB staff worker, for example, described a potential patient as "white faced, [with] a dull, tired look in her hollow eyes." Living in filthy conditions, surrounded by pale, starved-looking children, the woman was characterized by the staffer as a "border case mental defective"; this based on observation, not any cognitive testing, however flawed.[42]

As much as activists used eugenic terminology to describe individual patients, they did not use it as a category of analysis. They did not use or define terms like "mental defective" or the more catchall "unfit" in their reports. While they gathered detailed statistics on many aspects of patients' lives, they didn't test or estimate intelligence levels, nor did they record whether patients suffered from hereditary defects or deformity. They did not report on percentages of "fit" versus "unfit." Given their frequent use of the imagery, it is surprising that they made no effort to do so. Such figures could have strengthened their arguments, but their inability to secure this information underscores the difference between making sweeping statements about the unfit and in assigning actual people to these subjectively defined boxes. Such descriptions were more difficult to gather than data on race, income, education, religion, or nativity. The patient could not provide the answer, and the activist would have to assign them a category.

Despite their reliance on eugenic terminology and beliefs for propaganda, in the clinic, hereditarian eugenics took a back seat to environmental solutions for poverty. At best guess, more than 90 percent of clinic patients were eugenically "fit," which argues that the clinic was indeed dysgenic. Had the clinics held to a strict hereditarian view of eugenics, they might have targeted different neighborhoods for their clinics, measured hereditary traits, and likely offered sterilization for those constitutionally "unfit" to reproduce. Instead, activists treated "fitness" as a malleable category that could improve as health and material conditions were bettered. They treated women who had recently given birth and had not yet regained health, or those whose husbands were out of work. These problems were not innate, and given time, contraceptives, and good fortune, these patients' lives could improve to the point where they wanted more children. Until then, the savings earned with a smaller family made it possible for a mother to stay home instead of working in a factory, thereby improving her ability to care for her children and herself. Birth control, activists argued, helped to relieve poverty, one household at a time, by giving the parents more control over the timing of children and more options on how to spend their limited resources.

The Question of Race

While eugenic rhetoric was embraced by birth control activists, issues of race were generally shunned. Clinics did not do nearly enough to provide services to women of color.[43] It is ironic that the few efforts that were made have been tarred as racist plots to exterminate poor blacks, when the larger picture was one of neglect. By every measure used by activists to prioritize a woman's need for contraception—whether economic, health, or social factors—black women needed birth control more than white women did. But while activists rarely engaged in any discussion of race, most discriminated against black patients by denying them admission. When it came to extending clinic services to African Americans, these activists lacked commitment. While there were some notable exceptions, most suspected that African Americans did not want or would not use contraceptives successfully, or they hoped that African American women would take responsibility for organizing services in their own communities. As was demonstrated in the previous chapter, though African Americans found birth control a useful tool, it was not the most important outlet for their activism. With a few exceptions, this left African American women without ready access to birth control clinics.

The discussion of nonwhite patients in this chapter focuses on African Americans, who made up about 11 percent of clinic patients. Less than 2 percent of patients were Hispanic, often described as "Mexican Indians." Little has been written about pre-war efforts to bring birth control to Asian and Hispanic populations. Aside from anecdotal evidence that clinics in the Southwest and California saw larger percentages of patients from those backgrounds, much more research needs to be done to document how and when the birth control movement began to serve these minorities.

Birth control activists were not immune to the racism of their day. American society was steeped in racial thinking that divided and ranked people by both skin color and ethnicity, creating an idiosyncratic hierarchy that set Anglo-Nordic people at the top. Blacks, Hispanics, Asians, and other nonwhite peoples filled the bottom, along with the predominantly Catholic and Jewish whites from Slavic and southern European countries. With concern about immigration paramount in the early 1920s, clinic activists linked their efforts to "Americanizing" these newly arrived urbanites. While some questioned the ability of immigrants to use contraceptives responsibly, most Americans dismissed both African Americans and Hispanics as too "indolent" or "ignorant" to be capable of successful birth control.[44]

But as restrictive immigration laws were passed in 1917 and 1924, the flood of new immigrants was curbed and attention slowly shifted toward the "problem" of African Americans and Hispanics. As described by African American physician Dorothy Ferebee: "The public health problems of the Negro when measured by all health standards—mortality rate, morbidity rate, life expectancy, show the Negro to be in a most unfavorable position. The death rate is 50% higher than that of the whites, and 34% higher than that of the national average. The sickness rate is 43% greater; the length of life is 12 years shorter. Negro mothers die at twice the rate of white mothers, Negro babies at 2½ times the rate of white babies. Out of the one-quarter million Negro live births annually, 22,000 infants, or 9%, die before their first birthday, while an additional 18,000 are born dead, raising the total annual loss to 40,000 infants."[45]

Given the dire situation, the birth control services for African Americans were inadequate. In the 1920s, most African Americans attended a small group of integrated clinics in major cities (New York, Cleveland, and Pittsburgh). Over the next ten years, activists began setting up segregated services. The "Negro sessions" at Baltimore's Bureau of Contraceptive Advice were held one day a week from 1927 to 1937, after which a branch clinic in the city's northwestern section, staffed and supported by the African American community, was opened. The West Cincinnati Presbyterian Church Clinic divided its sessions into "white" and "black" days, while the Indianapolis Maternal Health Clinic set aside two sessions a month for black women. In

Houston, the plan was for appointments to be made for whites, blacks, and Hispanics on different days of the week.[46] More often, satellite clinics were formed. In Minneapolis, the local birth control league convinced the Phyllis Wheatley Settlement to house a "Negro clinic" in 1934. In Chicago, a clinic specifically for black women was opened at an African American settlement, the Abraham Lincoln Center.[47]

By the mid-1930s, birth control clinics began expanding into the South, though the process was by no means quick or certain. A hospital clinic was founded in Nashville's Meharry Medical School in 1935 by two African American physicians, Michael J. Bent and W. H. Grant.[48] In Louisville, a clinic for African Americans at the Afro-American Presbyterian Church was founded in 1936. Funded for three years by one of the board members of the Kentucky Birth Control League, it seems to have closed when the gift expired.[49] In 1937, clinics for African Americans were also formed in Birmingham (funded by Clarence Gamble) and in Miami, where the clinic was held in the home of an African American social worker.[50] Though there was a demonstrated need and interest in birth control clinics for African Americans, by the end of the decade the number of clinics that treated this minority was decidedly small.

While few activists discussed race and ethnicity in their brochures and propaganda materials, their actions revealed their attitudes. From the earliest decisions—where to locate the clinic, who should staff it, where they should advertise, and what groups they should lobby—race and ethnicity mattered. While many clinic activists may not have given conscious thought to the decisions they made, their biases defined the limits of the movement.

When Sanger founded the first birth control clinic, she did not locate it in Harlem, though the infant and maternal mortality rates and intense poverty there were comparable to the immigrant ghetto she selected. Sanger claimed she chose the Brownsville section of Brooklyn, populated largely by Italians and Eastern European Jews, because a delegation of women approached her for aid.[51] Another neighborhood she considered was New York's Lower East Side, also known for its overcrowded slums of Italian and Jewish immigrants. Choosing to serve white immigrants rather than the native-born African Americans was a decision that made Sanger's work harder, not easier. Putting a clinic in Brownsville meant that she had to hire an interpreter so that she could communicate with her patients. Treating Italians and eastern Europeans also made it more likely that the clinic would raise the ire of the local Catholic hierarchy, as priests saw their parishioners tempted by the clinic. In a pattern that would be repeated in the next twenty years, everything about the Brownsville clinic—its location, its staff, and its advertising—made it unlikely that nonwhite patients would attend. Brownsville did not ban blacks from attending, and in fact we do not know whether any black women attended, but it was set up to attract white immigrants from the surrounding neighborhood. Sanger linked nativist fears about the fertility of immigrants with a concern for the health of poor mothers and children, striking two pressing social topics of the times. She pitched the clinic in a way designed to win support from the middle class by addressing their fears of urban crowding and poverty, widely seen as problems that came with the millions of European immigrants to America's shores. The Brownsville clinic would teach immigrant families how to have smaller "American" families and to care for them properly, thus fitting into wider efforts to assimilate foreigners.[52]

While activists knew that African and Hispanic American communities could use their help, they prioritized whites, thinking that whites would make better use of the opportunity. These viewpoints were supported by eugenicists such as Raymond Pearl, who argued that because contraceptives required intelligence and foresight, whites were better suited to using them than African Americans. Pearl, probably echoing the beliefs of many birth control activists, argued that some more "automatic" method should be devised for African Americans because "the American Negro, probably generally and certainly under urban conditions, exercises less prudence and foresight than white people do in all sexual matters."[53]

These stereotypes led racists and eugenicists to fear that if whites used contraceptives while blacks did not, America's population and political structure could be fundamentally changed. For the Catholic demagogue, Father Charles Coughlin, it was an alarming situation. In his 1934 testimony against birth control in Congress, he warned that legalizing birth control would destroy the Anglo-Celtic population of the nation, reducing whites to a minority. Others turned this argument on its head. Marcus Garvey dissuaded African Americans from birth control, predicting that their high birth rates would eventually result in increased political clout.[54] Most women, black or white, resisted calls to increase their family size for such abstract goals.[55]

Activists who did not treat African American women found valid reasons for such neglect in the popular stereotypes of black women. When clinics admitted African Americans they questioned these characterizations. Describing African Americans as "cooperative to a marked degree," eager, and "enthusiastic" users of contraceptives, these clinics proved Pearl's assumptions wrong. Clinics in Baltimore reported "that Negro mothers are able to practice birth control just as successfully as their white sisters." At the BCCRB, they found "both Negro and white women learned and applied the clinic birth control methods equally well and with 95 percent success."[56] The challenge was not to develop a special contraceptive method for black women, but to figure out how to better deliver existing contraceptive methods to the black community.

But this was a challenge that few activists met. Though they left little to document their views about race, we turn again to their actions and find them reluctant to admit African American patients. Sarah Marcus, who was born and raised in the South and admitted holding racist views in her childhood, denied that Cleveland activists discriminated against African Americans: "I never never never had that feeling. I felt that they were sincerely interested in Planned Parenthood, that you should have your baby according to your own desires and ability to make the family circle a happy unit."[57] But there is some evidence that some activists had more empathy for white patients. In one instance, Little Rock clinic activists Raida Pfiefer and Hilda Cornish Coates suggested to their white domestic workers that they should attend the clinic, but did not invite their African American workers.[58]

Racist stereotypes of black women as lazy, ignorant, promiscuous, and vulgar were pervasive in American society, and it seems likely that many activists believed that African Americans had too many obstacles to overcome, even if aided by birth control.[59] Hints of racism among the white staff and organizers of birth control clinics can be found here and there in surviving records, but there are few sources where race is directly addressed. In Miami, Dr. Lydia Allen deVilbiss funded several groups of African Americans to start segregated branches of her Mothers' Health Clinic, but when they disagreed with her tactics she became deeply critical of their efforts. DeVilbiss was notoriously difficult to get along with, whether dealing with white or black activists, but her comments, calling the African American Miami clinic leaders "southern darkies" incapable of running a clinic without white help, are particularly crude. DeVilbiss pulled her funding and tried to sabotage the clinic's relations with the ABCL.[60]

Some activists blamed the prejudices of their white patients, some of whom complained about sharing waiting rooms and clinics with African Americans, for keeping black women out. In St. Louis, the Missouri Maternal Health Association found that "there was some resentment by whites at the Delmar

Boulevard Clinic where occasional Negroes are served." Their solution was to work something out with the Urban League to treat African Americans at local churches. In New York, some BCCRB patients were reluctant to attend the uptown branch in Harlem because it was in the "colored section." Sanger retorted, "I am not afraid of the patients either from the Bureau or from Harlem turning up their noses at Harlem provided it is kept clean."[61]

In large part, activists' inattention to African Americans fits in with the segregated lives that most Americans lived. While some white activists worked with African Americans, far more restricted their reform work, not just their birth control work, to helping underprivileged whites. They assumed African American philanthropists, African American club women, and specific organizations such as the NAACP and Urban League would take care of the black underclass. Few white activists considered questions of race when they created their clinics or showed any real interest or dedication toward racial justice or equality. When they imagined what their clinics would look like, the faces that they pictured, both in the waiting room and behind desks, were white. They saw integrating their clinic or developing a clinic specifically to treat African Americans, as a difficult and complicated undertaking. They probably felt less comfortable in African American neighborhoods. Instead of the gratitude they thought they should receive, many experienced distrust and hostility from prospective patients who feared that birth control clinics were part of a white plot to trick them into race suicide or involuntary sterilization.[62]

Activists treated African American culture as more foreign than that of the immigrant ghetto.[63] When white activists set up clinics in African American neighborhoods, they often created African American advisory boards, while those who set up clinics in predominately Italian, Jewish, or other immigrant communities felt no need to consult local leaders. Sanger consistently sought African American advisors when developing birth control services for blacks. Both with the BCCRB's Harlem Branch and the later BCFA Negro Project, Sanger established a consulting board to help her sculpt the birth control message for African Americans. This underscored her concern about the complications that race introduced to birth control clinics and the need for tailored propaganda for African American audiences. McCann suggests that such boards were brought in after the main shape of these campaigns were determined by whites, finding them somewhat condescending, but I find that these board members held more, rather than less, power over clinic policies than the boards of white clinics, which often served as rubber stamps for the clinic's officers.[64]

Race, more than ethnicity, gave activists pause. It made them crave an additional level of community vetting, or perhaps a buffer between them and their patients. Dr. Midian O. Bousfield, a black physician sent to observe the Harlem Branch of the BCCRB, described the problem he thought faced Dr. Hannah Stone. Stone, he contended, "was trying to work on one social problem (Birth Control) and suddenly found herself enmeshed in another (color or race). She did not have the patience to see it through." Though he found Stone pleasant and capable, her African American advisory council complained about her, and Bousfield concluded that "again and again white people, competent in every other particular get confused in the face of interracial endeavor. Lack of deep-seated interest usually accounts for this." The solution, he thought, was that black women should step up and take responsibility for promoting birth control among African Americans. Calling publicly, though in vain, for "some colored woman to become the Margaret Sanger of her race," Bousfield believed that birth control offered "the fine women in the race who are practicing medicine" an opportunity for a "remarkable field of endeavor, perfectly legitimate and ethical."[65]

The percentage of African American patients treated at birth control clinics nationwide in 1940 was slightly higher than found in the general population (12 percent of clinic patients were black, while only 9 percent of the American population was). Just as African Americans were clustered in some regions of the country, most black patients were seen in just a handful of clinics. Many clinics did not report their patient counts by race, which makes it difficult to determine whether or not they were integrated, but it appears that most banned African American patients. In some cases policy changes can be documented, such as when a clinic added a new location in an African American church or social service building, or when they set aside certain clinic days or hours for black patients. Sometimes it is only when an African American physician is hired that one can find out that black patients were being admitted. While none questioned that a white doctor might treat African American women, most found it unacceptable for white patients to be treated by an African American physician.[66] The clinics with the highest percentages of black patients were either in the South, where a segregated clinic, like the Birmingham Maternal Health Center, was the norm, or in the Midwest and Northeast, where the clinics were more likely to be integrated. Clinics in cities like Pittsburgh, Cleveland, Detroit, New York, and Indianapolis reported that one of every four patients was black.[67]

In the 1920s and early 1930s, African Americans had far more limited access to birth control than did white women. Not only did many clinics discriminate against black women, but the regions with the largest black populations had fewer clinics. Though the BCCRB and ABCL agitated for the creation of new clinics throughout the 1930s, they focused predominately on efforts to lobby women's groups and medical societies run by whites.

By the early 1930s, pressure to admit African American patients to existing clinics was slowly building. It came from two directions; from above, in the form of the national birth control movement, and from below, as African Americans sought services. In neither instance were these pressures strong enough to compel action, and in most cities apathy remained the norm. The Little Rock Birth Control clinic, which banned blacks, offers an example. In a city where one third of the residents were African American, no effort was made by white activists to admit black patients, or even to work with social agencies to develop separate black clinics. In 1931, the clinic's first year of operation, race was never mentioned at board meetings. In 1932, the board discussed a recent issue of the *BCR*, which had focused on African Americans and birth control. The June issue included an article by W. E. B. Du Bois, who argued that while African Americans were often encouraged to increase their population, it was the *quality* and not the quantity, that needed improvement. Birth control, he argued would help them to improve their quality. Fisk University professor Charles S. Johnson surveyed the state of Negro health, reporting on improvements in life expectancy and maternal and infant health, though all such improvements lagged far behind those gained by whites.[68] Most importantly for the Little Rock activists, perhaps, was "Clinical Service for the Negro," an article where Cornell sociologist Norman Himes questioned whether clinics were serving African Americans adequately. It also demonstrated the eagerness of blacks to have access to birth control. Surveying four urban clinics (Detroit, Cleveland, Cincinnati, and Baltimore), it concluded that in some cities African Americans were *more* likely to attend clinics than whites, and they "used the clinic as easily or more so than white patients." For example, in Detroit, African Americans made up 7.7 percent of the population of the city, but 25.2 percent of the clinic's patients.[69]

The criticism spurred the board to announce plans to open a special African American session that fall, pending funding. But four years passed without action. It was not until another outside impetus, in this case an offer of funds dedicated for the purpose, that the Little Rock activists began contacting African American physicians, public health nurses, and social work agencies to set up the service. Despite its professed commitment, for four years nothing had been done to make contact with the people who might have helped launch a black clinic. Serving African Americans was relatively unimportant to the board members; it was not worth raising extra funds, nor forging the necessary relationships with local African American activists and organizations. With funds practically dropped into their laps, Little Rock activists finally added a segregated session in 1937.[70]

At the very end of the 1930s, the BCFA finally sought to address the crisis in African American health care. As envisioned by Sanger, they would fund an effort to increase awareness of the health benefits of birth control among black doctors, social workers, and educators in the South. After the educational program was established, Sanger proposed that the BCFA help establish clinics and offset the costs of providing contraceptives to black women through public health programs. Dubbed "the Negro Project," this proposal was not at all dissimilar to the educational work Sanger's ABCL undertook with white women's groups in the 1920s. At that time the ABCL lobbied medical societies, social welfare groups, and women's organizations on the benefits of birth control and encouraged the establishment of clinics. The only difference in 1940 was that the emphasis would be on extending those efforts to African American groups.[71]

Sanger's plan relied on the cooperation of black leaders and would have focused on education and building grassroots support. But the BCFA's medical leaders wanted to shift responsibility for birth control to public health clinics, not develop the African American version of the independent clinic movement of the 1920s. Philanthropist Albert Lasker funded the project at a lower level than Sanger requested, and the BCFA proposed a different implementation. They wanted to set up public health demonstration clinics in a small area, determine how receptive African Americans were to birth control, and find the cheapest and most effective means of getting it to them. Sanger opposed this tactic, saying "It's all wrong. Every idea is childish been tried before and failed."[72] It was the BCFA proposal, however, with its medically controlled demonstrations, that Lasker preferred. As Sanger noted, the questions the BCFA proposed to answer had already been investigated by independent clinics in the 1920s and in North Carolina a few years earlier. Experience had proven that black women were just as eager for contraceptives as whites, that they used contraceptives with the same effectiveness as whites, and that birth control services could be added to public health work at a reasonable cost.[73]

As designed by the BCFA, the Negro Project consisted of two pilot projects in Tennessee and South Carolina. It funded field workers' salaries and contraceptive supplies in an effort to encourage the use of contraceptives. Though they created a Division of Negro Service to administer the project and gathered an advisory board of nationally prominent African Americans such as Mary McLeod Bethune, W. E. B. Du Bois, Walter White, and Adam Clayton Powell, control rested with white activists in New York and the white public health officers in the two states. Using a combination of visiting nurses (in South Carolina) and brick and mortar clinics (in Tennessee), the BCFA tried different methods of bringing birth control to the poor. In Tennessee, BCFA organizers worked in urban Nashville and developed tactics similar to independent clinics. Activists publicized the clinics to African American church leaders, physicians, social workers, and women's groups. Clinics were located in African American settlement houses at Meharry Medical School and Fisk University. Admissions were tightly controlled. Patients had to be screened into the clinic by visiting public health nurses. Women who heard of the service and wanted to use it had to secure the nurse's permission to attend the clinic. Of two thousand women who were referred to the Nashville clinics, only 638 women actually attended (32 percent). The BCFA reported that most women did not attend because they lacked transportation, suitable clothing, or child care. But it is quite likely that at least some of them were simply not interested. Even among those who attended the clinic, a majority did not stick with the program. Only 55 percent followed the regime "consistently and successfully." While this figure might seem low, it was on par with participation statistics from independent clinics that served a white clientele.[74]

In South Carolina, the BCFA aimed to reach women who could not travel easily to traditional clinics. A demonstration service was put in place in rural Berkeley and Lee counties, using the State Health Department visiting nurses. Nurses traveled into the hills, on dirt roads, and along rivers to identify potential patients. If the patient could not attend the public health clinic, the nurse secured foam powder contraceptives from the health officer and brought them to the woman in her home. The nurses instructed the patients in the use of foam powder and then returned periodically to check on progress. Any woman who qualified for public health assistance, whether black or white, was eligible for this service, and the racial breakdown of patients matched that of the counties as a whole (70 percent African Americans). The South Carolina program lasted almost two years, during which time 1,061 patients were "classed as prospects." Of those, 1,008 (95 percent) accepted foam powder and instruction and 840 (79 percent) reported "complete satisfaction." These figures are far higher than rates for independent clinics, and may reflect the lack of any viable contraceptive choices in this remote area. Any form of birth control was likely better than none.[75]

The Negro Project offers a mixed legacy. Once its educational component was stripped away, its focus was narrowed and limited. Because control over the project rested in the hands of white public health officials, it had little lasting effect among the people it tried to reach. African American doctors, club women, and social workers were not brought in at the local level to assist with these clinics. When the BCFA pulled out there was little infrastructure built to continue or expand the work. When neither Tennessee nor South Carolina agreed to fund the program after BCFA funding ceased, Planned Parenthood (the BCFA's new name after 1942) quickly lost interest. While they continued to operate a "Division of Negro Service" to increase awareness of birth control among African American organizations, much of the clinical work was left to the state and local leagues to operate. These were the same groups whose apathy had created the situation. Indeed, while the national organization continued to give lip service to their dedication to increasing African American awareness of contraception, not much had changed since the ABCL published its "Negro Number" of the *BCR* in 1932. While awareness of the need for birth control had been raised by 1944, the PPFA's African American field worker Marie B. Schanks described a movement that had not yet caught on with most African Americans. Schanks claimed that physicians and potential patients did not know about the birth control services in their localities, even if they might be more conversant with birth control itself. The PPFA was just beginning to forge relationships with major African American organizations, something it should have done far sooner if it were committed to actually helping African American communities.[76] Failing the emergence of a "black Margaret Sanger," extending birth control access to African American women continued to be a slow process, started and stopped at the whim of white activists.

Viewing birth control clinics through the prisms of race and eugenics reveals a different picture than what we see when we look at the national movement. While birth control activists may have embraced eugenics in theory, in practice they were less rigid, and certainly erred on the side of caution. And while the movement did not engage in overtly racist propaganda, many local activists made it extremely difficult for African Americans to take advantage of the reproductive choices that the clinics promised. Whatever the activists' personal beliefs about race may have been, there was no grand program to exterminate nonwhites or the poor. Race relations at clinics mirrored the relations in a given regional area. In cities where African Americans had few opportunities, clinics found it easier to close them out of their services. In larger cites, African Americans were sometimes able to consult the same physicians as whites and get the same services, but in only a few rare instances could they attend clinics in their own communities and be treated by black doctors and nurses.

There is no real argument about whether birth control activists wanted to spread their views on fertility to their patients. They did. But it is debatable whether they wanted to impose those views on an unwilling population. And the evidence shows that in almost every community, whether black or white, immigrant or native-born, women wanted birth control and attended the clinics willingly. Those who argue that clinics sought to exterminate the poor or African Americans ignore this crucial fact and instead make the argument that because the clinics were set up in certain neighborhoods, the inhabitants somehow had to attend them.[77] Patients were not nearly so naive or passive.

FIVE

The Clinic and Its Patients

In 1929, Margaret Sanger wrote, "Every woman who walks in that office seeking Birth Control advice is a victory not only for the Birth Control movement, but for the progress of women and a step for the improvement of the race."[1] The clinic's patients were as crucial to the success of the birth control movement as were the activists themselves. Without their interest and willingness, activists could not prove there was need and desire for contraceptives, nor could they prove that their methods were effective and safe. Helping women control their fertility was the reason for the movement. The experiences of the underprivileged women denied access to contraceptives either by law or economic realities were crucial to reforming law and policy. Activists used their patients' lives to personalize the propaganda, holding up examples of health, eugenic, economic, or other rationales for contraception. But these patients were real women—women with their own ideas, often strong ones, about birth control. Discerning consumers, they accepted the rhetoric of the birth control movement when it suited their needs and rejected those ideas that did not. They were sometimes dissatisfied with the clinic's advice, abandoning it and returning to older forms of contraceptives. But when the patient's goals meshed with those of the clinic, both got what they wanted.

Who was a typical clinic patient? Most were urban dwellers. Many were immigrants or the daughters of immigrants. Almost all were married to working-class men. Despite the activists' sometimes dramatic descriptions, most clinic patients were not destitute, and a significant number led reasonably comfortable lives. Most were in their twenties with only one or two children when they first sought aid, and most, though not all, were white. There must be more than demographic similarities, however. For every patient at a clinic, there were a thousand just like her who never made the journey. These few, perhaps just more determined than their neighbors, or fortunate enough to have a clinic nearby, were not satisfied with back-fence gossip, consulting drug store shelves, or poring over magazine advertisements. Whether they were poor, sick, or overwhelmed by the prospect of more children, contraception became a pressing enough need to fuel their sometimes heroic efforts to obtain accurate advice.

The depth of this need was dramatized by the 1916 Brownsville clinic in Brooklyn. Though the clinic had minimal advertising, almost five hundred women braved a trip to the storefront clinic in ten days' time. Some traveled from New Jersey or Connecticut.[2] By 1939, more than three hundred thousand more followed these first patients across the thresholds of clinics around the nation. Here, we will examine some of their lives and experiences, and explore the idea that the clinic offered working-class women more than just diaphragms; it offered a different way of looking at sex, marriage, and motherhood that had a profound impact on women's lives.

Piecing Together Patients' Lives

Few clinic patients documented their lives or experiences, so we must piece together their identities, motivations, and experiences through imperfect sources. These include letters detailing the dramatic events of patients' lives before attending the clinic—tales of multiple births, of frequent abortions, of grinding poverty, life-threatening illnesses, and marital discord. These depictions had purposes. Activists used them to secure support for the clinic. Patients created them to obtain help from the clinic. Both must be treated with caution and care. These are powerful descriptions that sometimes seem exaggerated, presenting "worst-case" scenarios of wretched women in desperate straits. There is no way to gauge the truth of any one story, nor can we extrapolate from individual stories about the lives of all American women. But because of the scarcity of first-person descriptions of married working-class women's lives, we should not lightly dismiss them.[3] To temper their emotional content, we need information from other sources. While statistical reports of clinics do not offer data on individual patients, they do provide a summary that enables both a corrective to the first-person narratives and a sense of how rare these cases were. Summary reports enable us to see trends over time, providing a norm against which we can gauge individual stories.[4] Another rare source of information reveals interactions between patients and activists, including complaint letters, letters expressing gratitude, and correspondence between clinic staff that discusses specific cases. These documents provide an unvarnished view of sometimes aggressive patients, not-so-sympathetic activists, and the tensions between them.

Chapter 2 discussed how clinic activists manipulated admission policies and clinic locations to shape their patient populations. They wanted to create the "perfect patient," a sometimes mythical woman who wanted birth control for all the right reasons, and whose plight was dire. Activists depicted these patients as inarticulate, pathetically desperate women, burdened with violent or troubled marriages, with hungry and ill-clothed children, in fear of another pregnancy. Victimized by circumstances before they even had a chance, they were unaware of wider opportunities and trapped in a downward cycle of poverty, large families, and a lack of education. Here you find stereotypes like Margaret Sanger's Sadie Sachs, whose death after multiple abortions supposedly spurred Sanger to take up the cause. For activists Dorothy Brush and Hortense Shepard in Cleveland, it was an anonymous patient at a prenatal clinic who drowned herself in Lake Erie rather than face a tenth pregnancy. As Sanger communicated to a reporter, "It makes your heart ache to hear their stories. . . . The women are so pathetically grateful, and so serious about it all. They are poor, hard-working women all of them, and they say they have such a terrible struggle to bring up the children they already have, that they cannot afford to have more."[5] In a particularly evocative example from her autobiography, Sanger described the despair of a woman denied access to the Brownsville clinic. The woman was just approaching the clinic as Sanger was being arrested and the clinic shut down. Sanger recalled hearing a scream: "'Come back! Come back and save me!' The woman looked wild. She ran after the car for a dozen yards or so, when some friends caught her weeping form in their arms and led her back down the sidewalk."[6]

How did it feel to be that woman, needing help badly enough to seek it from middle-class strangers, many of whom believed that the poor needed rescuing from their own failings? Activists depicted their patients' circumstances as grim, both morally and economically. New Jersey Children's Aid Society worker Jessie Condit depicted the slide of one factory worker with six children into destitution, despondency, filth, quarreling, and moral decline. Lengthy periods of unemployment had inured the family to the humiliation of asking for charity and their embarrassment about appearances prompted them to stop attending church. Their poverty necessitated that children work rather than attend school, but Condit believed that it also led to a lack of respect for their parents and the temptations of stealing and prostitution.[7] To Condit, this slide was inevitable given their lack of resources.

While social workers might emphasize the moral decay that accompanied poverty, the people who lived these lives saw daily life as a struggle to overcome material deprivations and a ruthless economic system that kept them down. "We are terribly poor," wrote an Arkansas woman to the Little Rock clinic, "We do not have enough to eat, never have milk. My husband is now a W.P.A. worker and has had no work for a year and a half. He has only drawn one W.P.A. check. Will you please tell me where, if possible I can buy whatever contraceptives that are safe and how much they cost. My doctor says he does not know. I do not think it fair to all concerned to have more children."[8] These women were suffering, but saw themselves engaged in a heroic battle to protect their children, provide a stable home, and comfort their husbands in the face of steadily dwindling resources. Writing to birth control activists or attending a clinic was one thing that a mother could do to ameliorate her situation. She saw her life very differently than Jessie Condit did, but they could both agree that no matter how the problem was defined, contraceptives could help.

How realistic was either of these portrayals? Both the patient seeking aid and the activist justifying her work had a vested interest in these gripping narratives of working-class life. Clinic activists wanted to create desperate "before" images in order to present successful "afters"—proof that the clinic had improved the patient's life dramatically. Patients hoped to secure treatment, and may have feared that without a dire home situation, they might be turned away. Perhaps they also needed to justify their actions to themselves as well. When contrasted with statistical studies of clinic patients, the stories in letters appear exaggerated, possibly even fictionalized. Indeed, Angus McLaren, in his *History of Contraception*, questions their veracity, arguing that letters written to birth control activists followed a known script that activists created through their propaganda.[9] The letters that survive have many common threads—an inability to afford a physician, a doctor who refuses to help, and failed early contraceptive efforts. But if the writer had the funds for contraceptives, consulted a helpful doctor, or found an effective method, she would have never have needed to write. The very act of writing to a well-known activist or organization on their chosen topic is bound to result in a selection of similar-sounding letters. Adding the fact that birth control organizations and activists would more likely keep or publish letters that supported their needs, we find similarities among the surviving letters easily explained.

But the letters vary as much as they coincide. Many betray an ignorance of birth control propaganda that I believe argues against McLaren's skepticism. Writers admitted having prior abortions and even requested help in procuring abortions. They freely discussed sexual maladjustments—an area that most activists shied away from in their propaganda, though it was often an important part of clinic work. If these letters were written to match the movement's propaganda, themes such as thwarted mother-love, eugenically unsound offspring, or extreme poverty should have predominated. In addition, many of the requests were quite straightforward—the writer felt no pressure to offer private details of her life. As compared to the average clinic patient, the letter writers probably represented the more extreme end of the spectrum. Clinic activists were more likely to save such dramatic letters for publication or use. Most women avoided these desperate straits by taking action earlier—attending a clinic, securing contraceptives, or obtaining an abortion.[10]

Clinic statistics tell a different story. You can still find the desperate cases—women in their thirties with eight or ten children—but they are outnumbered by younger brides with one or two children. Far from attracting women who were completely ignorant of contraceptives, those reports tell us that most patients had tried one or more contraceptive before attending the clinic. Statistics tend to flatten our image of patients into estimates and averages; they lack color and do not provide much information about motivation or patients' attitudes. Statistics also skew the analysis towards the experiences of patients from large, urban clinics, as activists there were more likely to gather and preserve statistical reports.[11] One serious drawback is that statistics were designed to answer the questions that activists wanted answered, not necessarily those that historians might ask today. For instance, interviews of new patients included questions about her sex life. So we know how often she had sex and whether she enjoyed it before she attended the clinic, but no one asked her how this changed once she was using reliable contraception. Likely, activists did not want to associate their work with increased sexual activity, even within the confines of marriage. Similarly, clinics tracked whether or not women continued using the diaphragm and whether it was successful, but did not ask patients whether they liked it, possibly because they had nothing better to offer.[12] Despite shortcomings, the statistical record presents a different view of patients, offering information we could not obtain from any other sources. Using both sources together helps temper the portrait of patients. What results is a more nuanced understanding of the range of experience.

There was not one generic patient experience, not even at the same clinic. Individuals brought different expectations, different attitudes, and engendered different reactions from the clinic staffs. Some patients were treated with suspicion by clinic workers. Some were rushed by harried doctors. Others were mothered, offered help to find jobs, money, or referrals to other clinics specializing in welfare or other health work. Patients responded differently to activists as well. While many were grateful for the help, others complained that clinic workers were paternalistic or nosy. Some simply had unrealistic expectations about the effectiveness of available contraceptives and about the amount of responsibility they needed to take in order to succeed. In short, patients were individuals—all seeking the clinic's help for the same problem—but for different reasons and with different experiences.

Demographics

Successful clinic patients were "determined contraceptors"—women who sought out the best contraceptive method they could find and stuck with it.[13] To be regarded successful by the clinic meant both that the patient successfully controlled her fertility using the clinic's method and that she attended the clinic regularly so her progress could be recorded. Conversely, an unsuccessful patient might be one who became pregnant using the diaphragm/jelly method prescribed by the clinic, or a woman who used the method successfully but never returned to the clinic, or even one who abandoned the method immediately.

Fertility and Family Size

Clinic patients may have been more fertile than the general population; they certainly were perceived that way. A forty-year-old mother of six described herself as "unusually prolific," claiming that no method had worked on her. A thirty-two-year-old mother of four claimed, "I am so easy to get pregnant," reporting at least five miscarriages, often only months after giving birth.[14] Some women may have described themselves this way to explain away what they feared was excessive sexual activity, claiming that they became pregnant nearly every time they had sex. Whatever was the case, it makes sense that such women would be more motivated than others to control their fertility.

In the letters written to activists, families of seven or eight surviving children and multiple miscarriages and abortions were common. Sanger described these women as "breeders," and guessed that they had a hereditary disposition toward motherhood, noting that they were "caught early and never released from the trap of involuntary motherhood." As one woman wrote Sanger, "I am one of the many who bear children too often. I love them dearly but I am only twenty-eight years of age and to give birth to my ninth child in about three weeks. Only have four living children, but they are winners." Or from another, "I was married when I was fourteen years old and now I am a mother of sixteen children, fourteen living and two dead and I am on my way for another child, three months."[15] An analysis of four thousand letters written to Sanger in the 1920s found that while the average writer had borne five children, one was the mother of twenty-five. One twenty-one year old had already borne eight children, on a pace for many more before her reproductive years ended.[16]

When we look at clinic statistics, such cases are less common. The statistical reports cover a far larger pool of women, and include all cases seen at the clinic. But there could be other factors at work. Abortions were more readily available in urban areas and 42 to 48 percent of New York and Chicago first-time patients admitted at least one abortion.[17] It is also possible that patients, meeting face to face with activists, might have under-reported abortions for fear that the activists would disapprove, either omitting the pregnancy completely or claiming a miscarriage. Women who wrote to activists miles away may have had fewer qualms. This might have led to more honesty, though without any likelihood of being caught, it could have encouraged women to exaggerate.

Twenty percent of clinic patients had six or more children. One patient claimed to have borne twenty-nine children.[18] The average was far smaller—between two and four children. Over the years, as patients' average age fell, so too did their family size. In 1929, San Francisco's Birth Control Information Center patients averaged 3.9 children, but by 1934 it was almost halved (2.1). In 1932, Pittsburgh's Maternal Health Center reported that

25 percent of patients had more than five children, while 40 percent had between three and five. In 1947 only 4 percent had more than five, and 22 percent had borne between three and five.[19]

These dramatic declines demonstrated a change in patients' reasons for using the clinic. Early on, the women were already in their prime childbearing years, between twenty and thirty-four years old, with families already growing. The longer a clinic operated, the more likely women were to hear about it even before they married. These younger patients tended to start contraception as soon as they were married, using the clinic to space the births of children over the course of a marriage.[20] The San Francisco figures confirm this, with patient age dropping as steadily as family size, from 30.6 years old in 1929 to 26.5 by 1936. By 1938, only 27 percent of patients in one New York clinic were more than thirty years old, and only 2 percent were over forty. Activist Carol Nash described the early days, when the clinic treated "the older, worn-out, thoroughly disheartened mother who had tried, without success, every method of birth control known to her. These mothers had already had so many pregnancies, so many miscarriages and abortions, that they begged to be relieved from childbearing. Gradually the older women ceased to be in the majority and we could discuss child spacing and family planning with our younger patients."[21]

Pittsburgh activists tracked the time between marriage and first clinic session, recording a decline from almost nine years in 1932 to just under four by 1948.[22] These observations and statistical studies demonstrate that as birth control became more accessible, patients adopted it earlier, using it tactically to plan their families.

Women who attended clinics successfully reduced their fertility. Whether they were trying to maintain their current family size or trying to space out births over time, 85–97 percent of patients were successful.[23] While we should not be surprised by this—it was a contraceptive clinic after all—it appears that even women who rejected the clinic's teachings experienced a decline in their fertility. In 1940, the BCCRB discovered that even if a woman reverted back to using condoms after attending the clinic, she was less likely to become pregnant than a condom-user who had never attended the clinic.[24] It appears likely that the careful explanations of the biology of conception and sex education helped women to understand that whatever methods they employed had to be used consistently. It may also have been that attending a clinic gave patients a sense that they could succeed, and offered them the support system to try.

Prior Knowledge of Contraceptives

Birth control activists portrayed their patients as ignorant of contraceptives, but this was simply not true. While there were undoubtedly women who had never heard of a diaphragm or who did not understand how conception occurred, this does not mean that they had never before tried to limit their fertility. Activists knew this of course, but they belittled the patient's research and past experience with inadequate methods. Clinics were invested in promoting one contraceptive method—the diaphragm. It was safe, effective, and woman-controlled, and to them these facts were more important than whether or not it was pleasant. In the matter of contraceptive choice, patients and activists had different goals and agendas. Many who "failed" as clinic patients simply decided that they preferred not to use the diaphragm. They did not necessarily reject birth control, or even believe that the diaphragm was ineffective. It just wasn't for them.

In 1925, 66 percent of BCCRB patients had tried some form of contraceptive before attending the clinic. By 1932 this figure had risen to 96 percent.[25] The most commonly used methods were douches (50 percent of patients), condoms (42 percent), and withdrawal (40 percent). Thirty percent of women had tried lactation (intentionally postponing weaning) and "holding back," (the belief that if a woman did not have an orgasm, she would not become pregnant). Twelve percent tried contraceptive suppositories.[26] Forty percent of these women had become pregnant using those methods, while others used methods inconsistently. This was especially likely with methods that relied on their husbands' cooperation (withdrawal or condoms). Some methods were clearly less effective: 70 percent of patients using douches failed, 60 percent of those using withdrawal or the safe period failed, and between 40–60 percent using sponges, condoms, jellies, and stem pessaries became pregnant. Diaphragms, used by a very small number of patients, offered the best statistical protection, with only a 28 percent failure rate.[27] No method was perfect, but some were clearly better than others.

Patients and activists had different outlooks on contraceptive methods. Both wanted an effective woman-controlled method, but they disagreed on the importance of aesthetics. Activists thought that effective protection was worth some discomfort or distaste. Patients put as much weight on qualitative factors as they did on effectiveness.[28] They could not afford, and most likely did not enjoy, undergoing medical examinations and contraceptive fittings. Most preferred products that could be purchased in drug stores or through the mail. Most avoided the stem pessary (an early intrauterine device) because it required a visit to the doctor both to insert and remove. As diaphragms also required a doctor's initial fitting, patients' wishes conflicted with activists' plans.[29] Ruth Robishaw's analysis of four thousand CMHA patients found that fully a third abandoned the diaphragm quickly. In Stix and Notestein's analysis of BCCRB patients, the numbers are even higher: 57 percent stopped using the diaphragm within two years of visiting the clinic. The most common reason was that it interfered with their enjoyment of sex. When pressed for more specifics, patients reported that they disliked the spermicidal jelly or cream that accompanied the diaphragm. They also said their husbands sometimes felt the diaphragm during intercourse and objected to it. Others claimed that diaphragms were too much trouble to use, while some found them frightening, distasteful, expensive, or offensive to their religious sentiments.[30]

Far from being ignorant and frightened, as activists portrayed them, many of the clinic's patients were educated consumers. As most had some prior contraceptive experience, they were able to compare the safety, effectiveness, and ease of use of the diaphragm/jelly regime to other methods. The breadth of their informal research could be impressive, as witnessed by one Arkansas woman's query: "I was told the salt water douche was reliable but it failed. Is the rhythm method safe and sure? I have been told that Lysol douches, permangenate or potash, etc. would do but I was afraid of them. Is the Lanteen Blue method sure? I heard of one case where it failed. Also how are the gold buttons and does one have to see a doctor each month with them? Would be very glad if you could help me by telling me some safe and sure method. I believe 4 or 5 children is pretty good for poor people."[31] No neophyte on the subject of contraception, this letter writer and others like her sought expert help to clarify information gleaned from neighbors, family members, druggists, doctors, mail order catalogs, advertisements, and birth control movement propaganda. Without access to birth control clinics, most women had no alternative.[32]

In sum, the women who attended clinics had an interest in contraceptives and had tried several kinds of contraceptives in the past, with unsatisfactory results. They may have wanted a method not yet available, the "magic pill" that Sanger dreamed of in the 1930s, something safe, secure, undetectable, and aesthetically pleasing. In lieu of that, some chose to make do with the methods they had already tried, while others would try the new method the clinic offered. It was not pleasant, but it was more certain of success.

Income

Birth control activists believed that all women wanted to control their fertility. The clinics were created to serve those too poor to afford a private doctor. They portrayed their patients as desperately poor, and indeed many of them may have been. But clinic patients were not among the poorest.[33] It is clear that "poor" meant different things at different times and in different regions of the country, which makes it fruitless to try to compare patients' income across clinics. In the Depression years, BCCRB patients had an average annual income of $1,250 in 1932, with a fifth of the husbands of the bureau's patients unemployed or only sporadically employed. In Arkansas, where per capita income was far below the national average, the husbands of patients at the Little Rock Birth Control Clinic earned between $260 and $364 annually in 1931–34. In Philadelphia, the average yearly wage was higher, at $1,352, a rate activists claimed was typical for unskilled laborers. But nearly half of the Philadelphia patients' husbands were out of work, prompting the clinic to treat 78 percent of its patients free of charge in 1931. Especially in the early 1930s, many patients' families were on relief or held WPA jobs. At some New York clinics the percentages on relief were high, ranging from 70 percent at the Recreation Rooms Settlement House Clinic (New York City) to 52 percent at the Monroe County Birth Control League (Rochester) in 1934. But at most clinics between 20 and 40 percent of patients were on relief, a characteristic of the availability of aid in individual localities as much as an indication of a patient's economic status.[34] Though the patients in most of the clinics were poor, they were not destitute.

When the economy began to improve in 1937, patient incomes slowly rose, but most would still be categorized as impoverished. In Massachusetts in 1939, clinic activists noted that at a time when it took an average of $27 per week to adequately provide for a family of six, 84 percent of their patients had to survive on less. In San Francisco, the recovery was not complete. The average monthly income of patients, $108 in 1929 ($1,296 annually), plummeted to $64.50 in 1932 ($774 annually), and by 1936 had only increased to $89 ($1,036 annually). As the decade came to a close, one could argue that while patients were not wealthy, fewer of them were in the very lowest economic categories.[35]

Most of the patients' husbands were unskilled laborers, from a variety of occupations. Many worked on farms, in factories, and as general laborers. In Pittsburgh, 70 percent of patients' husbands were laborers and only 15 percent were employed as white-collar workers. Between 88 and 97 percent of the patients themselves did not work outside of the home and relied on their husbands to provide for their families.[36] In contrast, the women who wrote letters to birth control activists were more likely to work; about a third worked outside the home as seamstresses, dressmakers, and factory workers, while others worked from their homes, taking in laundry, boarders, assisting their husband in his job or business, or doing farmwork.[37] Clinic activists argued that birth control promoted the more traditional family, with a bread-winning father and stay-at-home mother. They argued that when women could not control their fertility a crowded, impoverished home where women and children were pressed into work would result.

At most clinics, the economic criteria for admission barred middle-class patients from attending.[38] Some clinics did accept patients from more comfortable circumstances, though it was usually a small percentage—at the CMHA only 5 percent of their patients earned more than $50 per week. A few clinics, like the BCCRB and those run by the IBCL, encouraged middle-class women, using their fees to help subsidize the cost of treating indigent patients. These women believed that clinic doctors were both more knowledgeable than general practitioners and more discreet. While their middle-class patients might have been better educated than the rest, they resembled poor women in terms of their knowledge of and experience using contraceptives.[39]

As a rule, clinic patients were not wealthy, but they were not as destitute as activists portrayed them or as they portrayed themselves in letters written to activists. Most had to struggle to get by, especially in the early and mid-1930s, when massive unemployment made their lives more difficult than ever. While most patients paid some portion of the clinic's fee, the majority did not pay the full cost. Clinics adjusted their fees to take into account each family's circumstances and were willing to adjust these rates when those circumstances changed.

Motivations

Activists held that the key factor dragging women into poverty and despair was uncontrolled fertility. As Sanger described it: "Let us take a woman and a man starting out with an average man's wage of $12 a week. She is fresh and young, he buoyant and strong; life lies before them, and their desires are the best and their motives the purest. In a few years time nature has provided them, according to her laws, with a child every year, and they find themselves, in five years' time, with four little ones, living on the same wage that at first was only sufficient to keep two. Already her health is beginning to fail, although she may be only 23 years old. His strength is overtaxed by long hours of labor and the worry of extra mouths to feed."[40]

When a birth control activist looked at this vignette, she saw the mother's uncontrolled fertility as the immediate cause of harm; but when the same scenario was experienced by a patient, she likely put the blame on her husband's stagnant, insufficient wages. Regardless of the root cause, both agreed that birth control offered help. Of all the reasons that activists offered for birth control—economic, medical, eugenic, social, or feminist—patients found that economic reasons were the most pressing. In Little Rock, 81 percent of patients in 1931 sought help because they were poor, 15 percent because they were poor and unhealthy, and only 3 percent just for health reasons.[41]

Especially in the 1930s, when work was difficult to get and keep, any change in family status—a lost job, illness, or an unexpected pregnancy—could throw off the delicate balance between getting by and falling behind. As a twenty-three-year-old mother of three children, including one who died in infancy, wrote: "My husband is in bad health. He hasn't been able to work for five months. We were forced to move in with mother and father for the high rents that we had to pay. Some times I didn't even have enough for my babies to eat. Oh, how I cry to see my babies in this way. I don't know what I'd do if I had another baby that I know I can't take care of any more."[42]

Limiting births during times of financial distress was easier than securing a job or overcoming an illness when one could not afford medical care. Illness or incapacitation of a husband often led to destitution. In these cases, a woman had to earn some money to supplement the family income, and she could not become pregnant. As a Brownsville clinic patient told a reporter, "This is the kind of place we have been waiting for all the time. I have seven children, two are dead, and my husband is a sick man. Do you know how I got bread for them? By getting down on my knees and scrubbing floors for the baker, that's what I did when we couldn't pay the bill. Seven children . . . that's enough for any woman."[43]

Poverty led directly to poor health, and while it can be difficult to separate the two factors, 18 percent of the Little Rock patients listed health concerns as equal to or more important than economic motivations. Once her health was impaired, whether by malnutrition, disease, or overwork, a patient feared that another pregnancy could be life threatening. A thirty-two-year-old farmer wrote Sanger: "My health is very poor, I am nervous and just faint off sometimes before I can get to lie down. My heart has almost worried me to death yesterday and today, and it looks like everything the children do or say will run me crazy. My left side is paralyzed from no circulation and my leg is almost blue from the swollen veins, my ankle is blue and as large as two ankles ought to be. We are just poor people not able to hire help, borrowed $300 last year to make a crop, the drought caught us and we were not able to pay back a cent of it."[44]

Some medical conditions contraindicated pregnancy, regardless of economics. At the BCCRB, they found that about half the patients had gynecological or obstetrical conditions that made pregnancy risky, but another 40 percent suffered from kidney ailments, heart disease, tuberculosis, as well as general debility. Others reported hospitalizations, life-threatening complications from previous pregnancies, multiple miscarriages, and the deaths of their babies after a short time.[45]

It was much less common for women to come to clinics for social or eugenic reasons. At the BCCRB, only 7 percent of cases came because of family histories of birth defects, insanity, or violent or alcoholic husbands.[46] One woman, who described her pregnancies as extremely difficult, with stroke-like symptoms, fainting spells, and heart palpitations, confided: "Two years ago before this I had the horrible experience of having a monstrous birth and the next one was just like it. The doctors could tell me nothing of any value. Said I might have fifty more children and none would be like the last, or there may be more like it. Since I had two already now this leaves me in a very uncomfortable position as you can plainly see. These two little ones had no head, just a face, no skin or scalp on. The first was a seven months' baby but the other went nine months and was just exactly like it. My father is insane. Could this have anything to do with it? Our first three children are all right. I have three married sisters and their little ones are all right."[47]

A twenty-two-year-old mother of three reported what activists would call a "social" indication in a letter to Sanger about her husband: "He works, but spends it all in drink and cards, and when I tell him I must have some money he beats me and tells me to get out of the house. I would go only I wouldn't leave my children behind or if the baby was only old enough and could walk I would go but before I can raise them to come to that point I find myself in that condition again. Really I would rather die than have any more children because I have a hard time to have them and then my husband is a drunkard and a brute."[48]

Most patients wanted to control their fertility in order to better their economic circumstances or at least to prevent things from further worsening. As witnessed by their letters, many had difficult lives, plagued by ill health, troubled marriages, and a lack of resources. Gaining control over this one aspect of their lives offered them a hope that they could save a little money, regain their strength, or have some peace of mind.

Sex and Marriage

Birth control clinics offer a unique look at working-class women's sexual experiences. Most historical treatments of women's sexuality deal with middle-class women, and those that do explore the lives of the working class often tend to focus on single women.[49] Getting at the intimate details of the lives of these women is always difficult, but birth control clinics offer a rare source that argues that the changing sexuality documented by historians of middle-class women may have been delayed in the working class. Many clinic patients seem largely untouched by nineteenth-century arguments for "voluntary motherhood," which claimed a woman's right to refuse marital sex on the grounds of fertility control. Likewise, clinic patients seemed oblivious to the sexual revolution that began in the 1910s and 1920s and that encouraged women to demand their own sexual satisfaction in marriage. If the clinics' patients counted among the freewheeling generation of sexually active single working girls that Kathy Peiss described so vividly in *Cheap Amusements*, something happened to them after they donned a wedding gown, for most clinic patients revealed conservative outlooks on sex and marriage, virtually unchanged from those held by their mothers and perhaps even their grandmothers.[50] For many, sexual submission to a husband's desire was an unpleasant marital duty that could not be easily avoided. As one Arkansas woman wrote, "Any woman that loves her husband as I do mine wants him at home. And if a wife don't render due benevolence to her husband there is no doubt he will be out after other women and bringing home some bad disease sooner or later."[51]

Birth control clinics offered women not just a tool to reduce their fertility, but also a crash course in modern views on sex and marriage. Activists taught that marital sex should be frequent, desirable, and pleasurable for both partners, something quite alien to the experiences of many of their patients. Sanger blamed accumulated custom and prudery for the state of affairs: "For centuries women have been taught by custom and prejudice, especially in countries in which the Puritan tradition dominates, that hers should be a passive, dutiful role—to submit but not to participate. . . . Much would be accomplished if women were taught to be active, and men to check the tumultuous expression of their passion."[52]

I believe that the women who took such ideas to heart became successful clinic patients—attending regularly, committing to the methods prescribed, and using their contraceptives effectively. Women who resisted did not do as well. They were more likely to drop out or complain that the methods were too difficult or unappealing. Deeply ambivalent or even hostile toward the idea of more frequent sexual intercourse, some of these patients may not have really wanted an effective contraceptive if it meant more sex with their husbands. It is possible these patients, who adopted methods like continence, condoms, or withdrawal, may have done so as much to interfere with their husband's sexual pleasure as to reduce fertility. While the clinic removed the risk of pregnancy, it did nothing to make sex with their husbands more enjoyable. Hence, patients who disliked sex were also more critical of the clinic's methods of contraceptives.

Birth control and sex were inextricably linked, and some clinics used their unique access to their patients to gather information about the sex lives of the working class. The BCCRB questioned incoming patients about how often they had sex, as well as what was termed the patient's "mental adjustment toward sex relations." They found that their patients held many views similar to educated and middle-class women. Eighty-five percent of patients had sex between one and three times per week, on a par with the general population.[53] Only 7 percent reported having sex less than once per week. When asked to characterize their attitudes toward sex, 60 percent of BCCRB patients believed it to be "normal" and enjoyable, while 40 percent said they disliked it. Of those that disliked it, half believed they had minor difficulties adjusting to sex, while 40 percent reported feeling "dislike to the point of aversion." Ten percent labeled themselves as "frigid."[54] There is no way to determine whether these categories meant the same thing to the patients as they did to the activists who asked the questions. What seems clear is that most patients believed that their experiences were within the realm of normalcy based on their peer groups.[55]

Birth control activists were aware that many patients avoided sex, but they were less open to acknowledging that the reasons were more complex than a fear of pregnancy. Sanger repeatedly pushed the idea that if women were freed from the risk of pregnancy, they would embrace and enjoy sex with their husbands. This viewpoint was epitomized in a letter she received in 1924: "To me intercourse is so very, very repulsive . . . I have never cared for intercourse as a normal woman should, altho, before my first baby came, I did enjoy it. Six months before the second baby was born I began to grow nervous and irritable. I grew continuously worse, and became so dreadfully nervous when I even thought my husband wanted intercourse. When the penis touches me I felt as if I'd have to scream in spite of all I can do. We practiced total abstinence 3 mo. before the baby came thinking that afterwards I would be better, but it is just as bad as ever. I have no more emotion or desire than a child."[56]

Sanger argued that women were psychologically damaged by the fear of pregnancy, damning unreliable methods that were outside a woman's control, and the unreliable men who were more interested in their own gratification. Describing *coitus interruptus*, Sanger claimed that it was harmful to women because by the time the man withdrew, his wife "is under a highly nervous tension, her whole being is perhaps on the verge of satisfaction. She is then left in this dissatisfied state, which is far from humane. This does her injury." Sanger further advised, "A mutual and satisfied sexual act is of great benefit to the average woman, the magnetism of it is health giving, and acts as a beautifier and tonic. When it is not desired on the part of the woman and she has no response, it should not take place. This is an act of prostitution and is degrading to the woman's finer sensibility, all the marriage certificates on earth to the contrary notwithstanding."[57] Sanger's ideal marriage was one in which both husband and wife enjoyed sex without the fear of pregnancy.

While the fear of pregnancy was a factor in the sex lives of women, it was not the only reason women avoided sex. Many were at best ambivalent and at worst hostile toward it, as the practice was defined by and for the pleasure of the man. Historian Linda Gordon views this aversion as a rational reaction to an abhorrent situation. Activists faced with a patient who held these views needed more than diaphragms and jelly to change her outlook on sex. They needed to convince her that her marital life would become better if she overcame her sexual "problem."[58] In one such case, activists found "no recreation of any kind, healthful or otherwise, . . . the patient and her husband sit around the apartment all evening and he spends most of that time fondling her with the results that very early he insists upon retiring with her." The staff suggested that she bring her husband down for a consultation and that they try alternate sleeping arrangements. They advised her to have a frank talk with him, but internally doubted that she would oppose him in anything.[59]

In most instances, the clinic advised the patient to adopt her husband's ideas about sex, unlikely as it seems for such a woman-centered space. In *A Marriage Manual*, the guide written by BCCRB medical directors Abraham and Hannah Mayer Stone, frigidity is seen almost exclusively as a woman's problem, created by a lack of sex education and suppression of erotic feelings. Treatments included counseling and sex education that trained the woman to accept that her husband's ideas about sexual frequency were more "normal" than her own. When the Stones admonished husbands, it was for their insensitivity to their wives feelings, and selfish pursuit of their own gratification. Rather than counsel husbands to limit the frequency of sex with their wives, they advised them to be more considerate, engage in foreplay, and offer outward signs of affection.[60]

As part of their effort to provide birth control advice, activists delved into sex and marriage counseling. Cleveland clinician Sarah Marcus noted that while she was conducting pelvic examinations, women would start talking to her, "about impotence, their husbands, they'd talk to me about dryness of their vagina, they'd talk to me about the lack of orgasm and how to go about doing it differently."[61] At the BCCRB, staff dealt with a patient married for eight years "suffering from insomnia," who had never had an orgasm because her husband "erects immediately if he even kisses her once, and then has an ejaculation, and is unable to penetrate prior to ejaculation."[62] Activists listened to the complaints, like those of thirty-two-year-old "Mrs. M," married for fourteen years and distressed because her husband, who had formerly demanded sex twice per *week*, now insisted on sex once or even twice per *night.* Mrs. M., who admitted to "always giving in to him in everything," could not figure out how to return to their prior relationship.[63] In some cases, clinic activists even met with husbands to help couples work through their problems and enjoy better sexual relations. Again, at the BCCRB, staff taught "Mr. and Mrs. H." the basics of "erotic play," because Mrs. H. had complained that she had never experienced orgasm.[64] This kind of counsel went far beyond the provision of birth control, but it was critical to winning over the patients.

A majority of patients believed their sex lives were good. Fully 80 percent claimed that they experienced orgasm, with almost half claiming it occurred "usually," as opposed to "occasionally."[65] It is difficult to know whether to trust these responses, coupled as they are with other data that demonstrate the patients' ignorance about sex and their bodies. Patients may not have known what orgasms were, and might not have wanted to admit that. It may be that patients believed they should have orgasms, but one could easily argue that patients who thought that reports of a bad marriage might be more likely to get help might have exaggerated their sexual maladjustments.

Most patients described their husbands as "good," careful, or loving, but rarely happy. Uncontrolled childbearing put a terrific strain on marriages, especially when the wife's health was threatened by pregnancy. Even when couples worked cooperatively to avoid children, they felt the strain. As one woman wrote: "My husband and I have talked of giving up all sexual intercourse but you know how miserable that would make us. I could not do it. I would rather be dead."[66] Women whose husbands agreed to continence, or who practiced withdrawal, felt guilty that they were denying their spouses and worried that their husbands might become unfaithful or leave them. For the men, the fear of losing a wife to disease or the complications of childbirth or abortion kept them from having sex as often as they desired, or at all. Some exhibited physical symptoms—nervousness or despondency—while others became irritable and cross. As one woman described her husband's experience with continence: "He only says jokingly that he doesn't mind it much, and only revealed to me recently that he had been suffering seriously from his self-control for nearly a year. He is looking bad and I know this is injuring his health. I have great sympathy for him. We are both very young yet and he is healthy, and has strong sex desire, I can hardly stand to treat him thus."[67] Couples like these, whose marriages were founded on love and physical intimacy, benefited most from effective forms of birth control.

Not all husbands were "good," and activists found the wives of these men more difficult to counsel. The most common complaints were that men demanded sex too frequently, were unwilling to practice contraception, or were insensitive to their wives' desires and pleasure. Many were described as drunkards, wastrels, and abusers, who thought of their wives as replaceable breeding machines. Some claimed that they did not want more children but refused to participate in contraceptive efforts. Birth control activists were quick to blame husbands for these faults and criticized those who were unable to provide for their families. They blasted working-class men for failing to give their wives the attention and love they deserved, for refusing to limit their sexual enjoyment for the good of the family, and for abusiveness. Sanger described the "selfish husband" type, who, "like those natives of certain primitive tribes . . . have not yet learned to correlate, under the law of cause and effect, the sexual act and the birth of a child nine months later. Husbands of this type are imperative in their sexual demands upon the wife, and completely oblivious of the price that is exacted of her for their heedless moments of brute pleasure."[68]

As one woman wrote: "At the present time he has not spoken to me for three days. My heart is breaking. I keep away from him as much as I can and that makes him angry. I do nothing but cry and cry. He is so big and strong and I am so small. . . . I fear my husband so."[69] Another feared that her husband had a venereal disease: "He forces me to have intercourse whenever he wishes and will use no contraceptive measures, and I must have help. . . . To all my pleadings my husband turns a deaf ear. He beats me, curses me and deserts us for weeks at a time when I refuse intercourse."[70]

When husbands were truly uncooperative, violent, or incompetent, birth control clinics could offer only limited assistance. The practical advice they provided could help a woman whose husband refused to use a condom or practice withdrawal, because the diaphragm could be employed without a husband's knowledge or assent. At least, the clinic offered a place where women could tell their troubles to sympathetic listeners and receive suggestions or advice on other agencies to contact. In rare instances, it offered more than that. There are scattered cases of BCCRB and Little Rock clinic workers helping patients get away from boyfriends or fiancés, locate jobs or places to live, and in cases of marital discord, offering to counsel husbands about the maladjustments. While there is no evidence of activists encouraging women to leave husbands, it is not inconceivable, given their predisposition to the woman's plight, that they might have done so.[71]

Interactions at the Clinic

The actual meetings between patients and activists were rarely documented, but given the different values and ideas each held about contraceptives, sex, and marriage, there must have been tensions. The clinic's charitable setting placed a patient in the position of a supplicant, forced to answer prying questions in order to receive aid. It is likely that activists, wealthier and more educated, made them feel inferior. But the patient held some power in the relationship—activists needed her participation and would not needlessly alienate her. While activists seem to have had no trouble adding decorations and other external touches to make the clinics comfortable and cozy, there are some indications that actually interacting with patients was more difficult for them.

One of the central points of contention was the veracity of the data the patients provided, especially with regard to income. As seen in chapter 2, clinics did not investigate their patients, did not check to make sure they were married or that they had the number of children they claimed. But when it came to income, activists were more reluctant to take a patient's word. Some would investigate economic data, while others required referrals to verify the family's poverty. Patients who could pay for some portion of their care (usually the cost of discounted contraceptive jellies or the diaphragm itself) were expected to do so, but some activists believed the patient would lie about her income to save money. Most clinics relied on the honor system because they did not have the resources or the will to investigate their patients' financial backgrounds, but activists were wary of being taken in by a sad story.

The ways that clinics responded to patients who tried to cheat them reveal differences in the climates at the clinics, despite very similar policies. Sanger's BCCRB and the IBCL clinics offer a case in point. Both clinics had large numbers of patients, paying on an income-based scale. They supplemented these fees with outside contributions to support the clinic. The Illinois clinics were strict when dealing with patients. Effie Acheson Lyon, the IBCL executive secretary, suspected her patients' motives and honesty, advising other activists: "We have found that volunteer workers . . . are apt to let their sympathies get the better of them, and the women we deal with in the district are not slow to know this. We never refuse a woman for any reason, but often when in doubt of her story let her understand that we investigate our cases as to their ability to pay, and very often have found that understanding this the patient finds she can pay something."[72]

It is unclear whether the IBCL clinics actually investigated their patients, though they did employ social workers to meet patients in their homes. The main task was to encourage patients to return for scheduled follow-up visits, but they could also observe the family's economic condition. Compared to other clinics, the IBCL raised far higher percentages of their operating costs from patient fees, lending credence to the notion that they were more successful in collecting some fees from a majority of their patients. One of the settlement clinics, Medical Center number 5, reported that 80 to 84 percent of its patients paid for all or a portion of their supplies, even in the Depression years of 1935–36. The IBCL believed that this policy was crucial in building up self-respect, "As we have found that even in the poorest cases, much more value is placed on our advice if they can pay some fee, however small it is." From the patient's perspective, such a clinic came off as cold and suspicious. As one woman wrote to the St. Louis Maternal Health Center, "Neither do I like the atmosphere of the Chicago office, which of course has nothing to do with the price of jelly, but I could not help comparing it unfavorably with you in St. Louis, who show consideration and interest in every woman who found it necessary to come to you for help."[73]

If Chicago clinics were strict, Sanger's BCCRB was extremely lenient. Sanger herself was adamant that no woman should be turned away because she could not afford care. No investigation into the truthfulness of the patients' statements was made at the clinic; they were taken at their word. It was a policy that some activists found difficult, especially in the throes of the Depression, when the numbers of patients too poor to contribute funds rose dramatically. Caught between the patients' plaintive stories and the clinic's shaky finances, BCCRB staff found themselves in the situation of Marion Frances Warren, a worker stricter than most, who was accused by patients of unfriendliness. Warren defended her actions by offering a list of instances in which patients were abusing the clinic's kindness. She ticked off examples of women who tried to "put one over on the clinic," arguing that those who could pay something ought to be asked to do so. She described "Mrs. H.," who had attended the clinic with four friends and returned to complain that she had been charged more than her friends for the same service. Mrs. H. claimed that she had told the truth about her husband's income while her friends had lied, and on questioning, the friends admitted it and increased their payments. Warren described the case of "Mrs. R.," who had tearfully explained that she had only a few cents to last until the next pay day, but later, in the supply room, forgot her story and offered to help Warren change a ten-dollar bill, opening a purse with fifty-one dollars in it. According to Warren, Mrs. R. admitted that both she and her husband were gainfully employed and agreed to pay the balance on her account that day. "Mrs. S." had come to the clinic with a husband out of work for nine months, claiming to have been referred by a social agency for free care. Warren was suspicious because the agency usually sent written referrals. On calling the agency, she found that the S. family was known as one that always tried to trick social work agencies, and that Mr. S. had been employed at a good wage for two years. Warren feared that when such patients secured free treatment they would "spread the news all over the neighborhood." Warren's behavior resulted in complaints and her eventual dismissal, but in many clinics her dedication to insuring that the clinic gave free care only to those who really needed it would have been seen as admirable.[74]

Perhaps what is at work here is a different perception of the clinic's function. In Illinois and in Frances Warren's mind, the clinic was a charity, and as such, they wanted to ensure that the patients deserved its services. The view was that while a clinic worker might be sympathetic to the plight of the women who came to their doors, she need not suspend her critical faculties. With limited resources, the IBCL needed to raise as much money as possible from those who *could* pay to subsidize those who could not. Activists like Warren, it could be argued, wanted to make sure that the clinic could provide free care for the most "deserving" people possible, and in order to assure that she would press patients to pay as much as they possibly could. The reason that we know of Warren's actions is because patients complained to Sanger about her behavior. We don't know what they said to Sanger, how Warren actually treated them, or what their versions of the events were. Could those patients actually afford the fees as easily as Warren assumed? Did they find it embarrassing to be questioned by openly suspicious staff members? Even if one assumes that Warren described the interactions accurately, her confrontations alienated the patients. And that was something that Sanger was not willing to risk. For her, the clinic was less a charitable enterprise and more a means to advance the birth control cause. Alienating a patient who could afford to pay some portion of her fee was just not worth it to Sanger. Though similar records are not available for most clinics, it is my belief that the BCCRB was likely an anomaly in this regard. It was wealthy enough to be able to offer more free care than other clinics and its goals were broader than just providing services to its patients.

Rare instances survive in which BCCRB patients criticize the care they received. In 1929, a forty-year-old mother of six complained to Sanger that she had become pregnant twice in seven months while using the diaphragm as prescribed by a bureau physician. She paid fifteen dollars for her treatment and claimed that she was promised 100 percent certainty if directions were followed intelligently and faithfully. Sanger responded with a sympathetic letter, urging her to return, and explaining that while they could not guarantee that a patient would never become pregnant, they had a 98 percent success rate. Sanger ordered an investigation of the case, and found that the patient had failed to return for her follow-up visit as the clinic recommended. Instead, she had waited two months (after her first pregnancy ended in a miscarriage) and was then found to have been inserting the diaphragm upside down. Hannah Stone noted that the patient suffered from fibroid tumors, and wondered whether she had actually been pregnant at all. Because she used the method incorrectly, the BCCRB refused to accept blame, but their tone in dealing with the patient was conciliatory and encouraging. Sanger invited the patient to return to the clinic after her baby was born, promising to go over the use of the method with her personally.[75] Another patient who visited the BCCRB's Harlem Branch believed that the medical examination she had received had caused her to develop appendicitis: "During the examination with her hand, I believe, in the vagina, she pressed against my appendix with vigorous pressure. I felt pain and winced and my muscle contracted, she pressed hard again and I suffered the same reaction, She smiled and said something to the effect, 'That hurt, didn't it?' I said it certainly did. She gave me the information and assigned the reason as chronic appendicitis."[76]

The patient reported feeling weakness and pain after the visit, was unable to make it to her follow-up visit, and when a clinic worker phoned her she reported her problem. She was advised to keep the BCCRB informed; she consulted a physician, reported that she had appendicitis, and underwent an operation. Sanger commiserated, saying she was "sick at heart" over the patient's condition and thankful that the operation was successful. She asked Hannah Stone to delve into the records and Stone discovered this was not the first complaint lodged against the doctor, leading her to muse, "What it is, I don't know, but it certainly makes a very bad impression on sensitive persons. I think myself, that [the doctor] is inclined to be neurotic and I think we should get rid of her." Sanger assured the patient, "I have taken steps and shall continue to make as certain as one possibly can for the future that caution and gentleness shall be an outstanding feature in the technique of any physician connected with our work hereafter." She again invited the patient to return to the clinic when she was fully recovered.[77] This focus on patient relations was certainly unique for a clinic that dealt mainly with charity cases.

A successful clinic provided a useful service to its patients, with minimal red tape and maximum sympathy, something patients did not always experience at other social service and welfare organizations. Clinics did not use strict morals or means tests to determine admissions, nor did they stigmatize extremely poor patients or those with large families. Patients did not want to be interrogated about their finances and ability to pay; they wanted a contraceptive that was both foolproof and pleasant to use (even if it hadn't been invented yet). Clinics had to walk a fine line between catering to their patients' desires as one might do in private practice and running a charitable service that both kept an eye on its bottom line and gathered the data needed to justify its existence. That patients and activists had different ideas about the shape clinics should take is revealed clearly when the Pasadena Hospital sought advice on how to increase attendance. Patients wanted to do away with strict appointments, adjust hours to coincide with a well-baby clinic held there, loosen admission requirements to allow married women to attend for economic reasons, and gather only "pertinent" information about the patients. These improvements were all about how the patients were treated and how easy attending the clinic was for them. When the hospital asked doctors and social workers for their opinions, they focused more on structural improvements in the clinic's outreach: conducting more follow-up checks on patients, increasing publicity to social agencies, making referrals easier, and appealing to men through lectures. Each stakeholder in the clinic had their own perspectives and values.[78]

Sanger acknowledged a "new generation" of patients, who did not want to answer questions about religion or income levels.[79] Noting that paying patients "think we should not ask questions that a Dr. in his office would not ask," Sanger was willing to sacrifice some data-gathering objectives in order to retain patient loyalty and goodwill. She decided to stop asking patients about their religion, and decided that economic questions would only be asked if the patient sought a reduced rate.[80] But Sanger's position was unique. Many more activists, like BCCRB manager Marjorie Prevost, believed, as did many social workers of the time, that clinics were engaged in uplift work and that part of their mission was to train the poor to avoid the "degrading effect of pauperization."[81]

Clinics that became a part of their neighborhood community were more successful in attracting and keeping patients. In Georgia, a clinic attracted African American patients by pitching itself as a social club. In Houston, activists' work with African American public health and school nurses resulted in crowded sessions.[82] Those clinics that refused to take into account the needs and desires of their patients withered from a lack of interest. This can be seen most clearly in the hospital clinics sponsored in New York by the CMH. Patients believed that their reasons for desiring contraceptives were second-guessed and devalued and that the clinic was overly regimented and complicated. As a result, few attended.[83] In other instances, while patients might have been initially uncomfortable entering the clinic for fear of gossip or rejection, after a short time they referred friends and family to the clinic, unafraid of any perceived stigma. As Lenore Guttmacher remarked about mill town organizing, "At first it was difficult to break down the apathy of the women. They do things in groups and are tremendously influenced by each other. But once one of the leaders or popular women have come to the clinic with me, the others start following."[84] Sisters, neighbors, mothers, and friends were the best advertisements that the clinics had, and provided the best evidence that despite intrusive questions, naive assumptions about working-class life or marital relations, and the "do-gooder" mentality of the activists, patients thought that the clinic offered enough value to refer their friends over and over again. One daughter gave her mother the cost of travel to the St. Louis clinic for a Christmas present; in another case a group of neighbors chipped in to buy "decent" clothing for a friend with ten children who was too embarrassed to attend the clinic wearing what she had. In Los Angeles, one happy patient promised to "bring you every woman on the street who is sick," by saying, "Look at me, see what the Mother's clinic has done for me and my eight children. They will help you too." Clinic workers from Sanger on down rightly saw these referrals as an approbation of their work, for, as Sanger wrote, "No woman would recommend another to go for treatment which she had found a failure."[85] Missouri's Maternal Health League reported on the importance of these "missionary" patients who, after receiving care, "gladly tell others" and build up confidence in the clinic until "new patients present themselves fully convinced of the adequacy of our method and some of the skeptical older patients return on their own initiative to try again."[86]

In 1931, Marie Kopp reported that 48 percent of BCCRB patients were referred by other patients. Welfare groups (social workers, doctors, and nurses) referred only 32 percent and birth control publicity (ads, cards, newspaper articles, and lectures) were responsible for 19 percent. Despite the fact that activists actively encouraged referrals from welfare groups, by 1938 Dickinson and Morris reported that 47 percent of referrals came from other patients. Social agencies were responsible for 29 percent, physicians for 10 percent, and publicity for only 8 percent. Despite their efforts to increase referrals from these professionals, it was word of mouth among the patients that remained the driving force behind the clinics.[87] While many such clinics were able to create a pleasant atmosphere, only some were skilled enough to get information from the patients without making them feel uncomfortable. For women attending such a birth control clinic, the experience was positive, one in which they felt not only that they were getting needed help, but that they had entered a community of women with similar goals. As one Los Angeles patient described it: "I did go to the Clinic and they are splendidly helpful beyond the mere dispensing of advice and materials. They are very, very careful and keep records of every little thing in connection with the case. This I have to say about the clinic. The spirit is most admirable. Prince or pauper need not complain. There is a feeling of at-homeness when one enters, growing more and more as woman's knowing heart reaches out to help those who want to know. They are very careful not to let anyone feel beneath them. Their helpfulness cannot be compared with the pauperizing attitude of some charity clinics."[88] In addition to practical help, clinics provided patients with someone to talk to about their problems, someone who, despite her class and education, was there to listen. A Brooklyn clinic worker reported that, "Into the ears of the women in charge are poured the most heart-rending tales of mental and physical torture from women whose health has been wrecked through excessive childbearing and overwork." Patients in this state, according to ABCL organizer Henrietta Hart, had "suffered too intensely; they had lost all false modesty. They had passed through the worst, and hope of salvation was almost more than they could grasp."[89]

Hundreds of thousands of American women of all races, religions, and ages came to birth control clinics. There they found a very different outlook on marriage, sex, and a woman's role and potential. Many passed through the clinics briefly, returning to whatever contraceptive they had been using in the past, but many more stayed. We know that they were able to reduce their fertility, in some cases dramatically, with the knowledge and training they received. But we can also speculate on what else might have happened at the clinics. Most patients probably picked and chose among the messages that the birth control activists offered, just as they selected and abandoned their contraceptives. Some were undoubtedly changed by the experience. Rose Halpern, one of the original Brownsville patients, was moved to testify at Sanger's trial in 1917, "as a demonstration of the need of information on birth control among the poor." The wife of a garment worker with six children, she founded the working-class birth control discussion group, the Brownsville Mother's League. Seventeen years later, she had borne only one more child, and on Sanger's behalf traveled to Washington to testify before Congress against the Comstock Act, dramatically shouting to the assembled congressmen, "I could decidedly say Mrs. Sanger saved my life."[90]

A national survey in 1938 reported that 79 percent of American women approved of contraception. Few of them ever attended birth control clinics.

Only an estimated 239 out of every 100,000 women in the country (0.2 percent) entered a birth control clinic in the 1920s and 1930s.[91] Many simply had no access, for despite the boom in clinic openings, there were never enough to cover every city or town. Many women obtained contraceptive advice directly from their physicians, from druggists, or from mail-order catalogs. Others continued to rely on older preparations, vinegar douches, sponges, and other household items, or were willing to continue using abstinence, withdrawal, or the increasingly publicized rhythm method. Those who turned to the clinics were the "determined contraceptors," the women who for many reasons made an extraordinary effort to control their family size.

At the birth control clinic, women found both sympathy and expertise. Though clinics were certainly not perfect, in them women found other women, some wealthy, some medically trained, who would listen to them, help them, and provide them with information they wanted. Working-class women were given a forum to talk about their home lives, their marital relations, and their sexual feelings. For the first time in their lives, many patients received the attentions of doctors and referrals to other medical services when needed. Most of this advice was given freely or at low cost. They found education as well, about their bodies, and in some cases about the way their marriages and lives could work. Clinics gave women a space where they were treated like responsible individuals—in charge of their bodies and their family size—and this may have enabled them to take the messages of maternalism and freed sexuality into a new era, one in which they could conceive of a different path for their lives or for their daughters' lives. For the middle class these messages were conveyed through public campaigns for birth control, a message made more compelling by the economic crisis of the Depression. For the working class, the expense of obtaining contraceptives slowed this transition and the birth control clinic served a critical role, on a patient-by-patient basis, providing those fortunate few with the information that every woman needed to know.

SIX

Clinics and the Federal Government

In 1938, an exasperated Margaret Sanger complained that, "When the matter is put up squarely to government officials who should properly inaugurate birth-control services on a nationwide scale, we run into an impenetrable wall of inertia and subterfuge."[1] Activists created independent birth control clinics to fill a void left by the government, organized charities, and the medical profession, but efforts to secure federal funding for birth control ran aground on the shoals of both moral and medical opposition. The 1873 Comstock Act classed contraception as an illegal obscenity, but because the act was limited to the mails, it did not criminalize birth control clinics. It did make them harder to operate. The law restricted a clinic's ability to contact patients, garner publicity, and secure supplies. While such practical obstacles could be overcome, they left a moral taint that linked birth control with illegality and immorality.

The medical obstacle was more general. The government was reluctant to take any practical responsibility for its citizens' health. Two government agencies, the Children's Bureau (CB) and the U.S. Public Health Service (PHS), charged to improve the health of women and children, could have spearheaded government-funded contraceptive clinics, but neither provided direct medical care. The doctors who ran the PHS rejected clinics because they opposed "socialized medicine" as a threat to private practice. The social workers at the CB feared that birth control's moral taint would complicate their mission and threaten the small gains women had made. Shunned by two reluctant partners, birth control activists were forced to dance alone.

The relationship between the state and birth control was a critical one for the clinics. Independent clinics were only a stopgap. Activists could not privately fund the number of independent clinics needed to provide national coverage, especially in rural areas. Federal opposition to birth control stymied the efforts of birth control activists who lobbied the government in the 1920s and 1930s. After more than two decades of agitation, activists had achieved little. The Comstock Act stood, birth control was still categorized as obscene, efforts to secure federal support had failed, and those clinics that were supported by government funds treated only a tiny percentage of clinic patients.

Clinics and the Law

The legal victories won by the birth control movement had little impact on the operation of clinics, where state law and the threat of local prosecution were the critical factors. The national birth control movement's focus on changing the Comstock Act was designed to make a symbolic statement and to encourage the repeal of the many "little Comstock Acts" that had been passed in individual states.

The Comstock Act was rushed through Congress in 1873, on the strength of Anthony Comstock's anti-vice campaign. This law criminalized the mailing of obscene material, specifically banning contraception, abortion, and other "lewd, lascivious and filthy" materials.[2] The law was inclusive, banning the devices themselves as well as information about contraception and where one could learn about it.[3] Nineteenth-century prosecutions focused on published works and mail-order contraceptives. Though created to stifle contraceptives, the Comstock Act had the opposite effect. In 1913, the United States Postal Service suppressed an article on venereal disease, and in 1914, a radical feminist journal that included articles mentioning "birth control." The author of that article and the editor of the journal, the *Woman Rebel*, was Margaret Sanger. Not content to pay the fine and agree to abide by the law, Sanger challenged both the federal and state Comstock Acts by publishing and distributing illegal pamphlets like *Family Limitation* (1914), and by launching a movement to change public opinion on birth control and to lobby state and federal legislatures to overturn the bans. Sanger won legal victories in 1918 and 1936 that secured the right of physicians to prescribe and mail contraceptive material for health reasons. Perhaps more importantly for the clinics, her publicity campaign made prosecution under existing laws less likely.[4]

In the 1920s, legislative efforts to overturn the Comstock Act divided the birth control movement into two hostile camps. One, led by Mary Ware Dennett and the Voluntary Parenthood League, sought to remove contraception from the Comstock Act's list of obscene articles (leaving abortifacients and items leading to indecency and immorality). Dennett's goal was to allow anyone to provide birth control information or materials. While the "open bill" was attractive to many activists because it removed the stigma of obscenity, it did not prevent quacks from promoting dangerous methods. Opposed by both doctors and legislators who were uncomfortable with any discussion of sex or birth control and generally hostile to women lobbyists, Dennett's effort floundered in the mid-1920s.[5]

Sanger's perspective on repeal was more limited and pragmatic. She associated birth control with public health and medicine, and her approach, backed by the plaintive cries from worn-out mothers, was that birth control would benefit society. She was able to add the voices of doctors, sociologists, economists, and clergymen to those of the lay activists by promoting a "doctor's bill." Sanger's legislation sought to remove medical professionals from the act's ban, arguing that birth control was a medical issue that would reduce maternal and infant mortality and improve health, economic stability, and eugenic "fitness." She faced heated opposition from Catholics, doctors, and legislators, but by the mid-1920s Sanger's campaign was the only viable option and by the late 1930s she succeeded in securing a judicial victory.[6] By that time Sanger sought to join birth control's star to the burgeoning public health movement. She and other activists encouraged states to view birth control as a tool to reduce welfare and relief budgets. Linking social scourges like crime, mental illness, prostitution, abortion, and delinquency to the inadequate parental supervision and love of "unwanted" children, activists touted the lasting effects of smaller families—first on the family, and then throughout the community. When making these arguments, birth control activists seized on problems that the government had already agreed to address, like infant and maternal mortality, and demonstrated how birth control could alleviate them.

Most interpretations of the Comstock Act's impact on birth control fall into two categories—studies that focus on the impetus for the creation of the act in the nineteenth century, and legal histories of the incremental repeals of the twentieth century. Works like Janet Brodie's *Contraception and Abortion in the Nineteenth Century* define the situation faced by twentieth-century activists, but end their stories there. General histories of censorship treat birth control only incidentally, and usually focus on a few major prosecutions. This "big case" mentality views the birth control movement through its victories in *State of N.Y. v. Margaret Sanger*, the *U.S. v. One Package*, and the *Griswold v. Connecticut* cases. Most scholars have focused on Connecticut and Massachusetts, states where laws were more restrictive and prosecutors more willing to bring charges. Very little work has been done on the law's impact on clinics, and when it is discussed, scholars often place too much emphasis on certain cases, such as the 1919 appellate decision on the Brownsville clinic, regardless of the fact that it only affected New York.[7]

In 1937, fresh from their U.S. Circuit Court of Appeals victory over the Comstock Act with the *U.S. v. One Package* case, birth control activists crowed that the victory cleared the way for the accelerated establishment of clinics. They argued that before the decision, physicians could not legally obtain supplies and information, a situation that impeded research. Historians accepted their interpretations, arguing, as Alvah Sulloway did, "After these decisions, the door was opened to a nationwide advance in the establishment of clinics, to widespread publicity about birth control, and to the active support of the medical profession." But clinics were expanding rapidly before the *One Package* decision, contraceptive research was flourishing, and birth control activists had decided to flout the law. All of which makes it difficult to argue that the Comstock Act had a great impact on clinic work.[8]

Starting with her prosecution in 1914 and through her continued disdain for the act, Sanger exposed a flaw in the government's war against obscenity. With Anthony Comstock's death in 1915, prosecutors were less eager to prosecute obscenity charges, including birth control cases, because the public had lost interest. For example, when the once-feared New York Society for the Suppression of Vice launched a "clean books" campaign in 1923, its effort to strengthen obscenity definitions backfired, as vocal and powerful opponents organized against their campaign. While attention focused on censoring magazines and movies in the 1920s, the courts adopted more liberal interpretations of obscenity, as seen in rulings on James Joyce's *Ulysses* and Mary Ware Dennett's *Sex Side of Life*. In many cases, these rulings excluded medical texts discussing issues like birth control.[9] Though it was widely known that Sanger and the ABCL regularly mailed illegal birth control materials, including Sanger's pamphlet *Family Limitation*, prosecutors refused to indict her, unwilling to provide her with free publicity. In 1926, when Sanger's husband J. Noah Slee tried to have his contributions to the ABCL declared tax exempt, he set off a protracted dispute with the Internal Revenue Service. In the course of the investigation, evidence was gathered proving that the ABCL broke the law by mailing *Family Limitation* and clinic directories. The proof of illegal activity should have doomed Slee's contention that it was a charity, but despite his lawyers' fears, neither Sanger nor the league was charged with violating the Comstock Act.[10] Even when the government did prosecute birth control cases, as in the example of the Italian anarchist Carlo Tresca, the Comstock Law was used as an excuse to incarcerate a man identified as anti-government.[11]

Because birth control clinics generally provided contraceptive information verbally, the federal Comstock Act had no jurisdiction over them, though state laws were often written broadly enough to limit their work. But the Comstock Law did more than keep the mails free of contraceptives; it left a shadow over almost every aspect of a clinic's work. Clinics and leagues could not advertise in newspapers, circular letters, or magazines; they technically could not provide addresses for their clinics in anything that might end up in the mail. Contraceptive manufacturers could not legally ship diaphragms, jellies, ointments, or instructions to clinics, making it difficult to stock supplies.[12] Even if the law was not often enforced, clinics were vulnerable to prosecution. As Sanger recognized early on, the Comstock Act's key impact was the stigma of obscenity and immorality that it attached to birth control. Added to that was the public's hazy understanding of the specifics of the law, which left doctors, scientists, educators, and some birth control activists uncertain about birth control's legality. When faced with this confusion, many physicians, social workers, and scientists took the easy path of refusing to have anything to do with it so long as it remained illegal.

Efforts in the mid-1920s to secure a free-speech repeal of the Comstock Act were followed by the more sustained effort to pass Sanger's "doctors-only" bill, pushed by the ABCL, and after 1929, by the NCFLBC.[13] But after nine years of lobbying in Washington, during which the NCFLBC drummed up a tremendous amount of grassroots support, Sanger had only secured a few congressional hearings. Her bills were quietly killed in committee and only one ever came to a vote, was passed, but was then called back on a technicality. After 1935, Sanger faced facts—the power of the Catholic lobby made it unlikely that the Democratic White House would support her bill, and she admitted that the chances of amending the Comstock Act were slight.[14]

Instead, Sanger pursued a judicial decision. In December 1936 the *U.S. vs. One Package* ruling interpreted the Comstock Act as if her bill had been passed. The decision, on a case where Dr. Hannah Stone imported pessaries from Japan, held that contraceptives should not be banned when mailed to or from "conscientious and competent physicians for the purpose of saving life or promoting the well being of their patients."[15] With victory in hand, Sanger and other activists suspended their legislative work and disbanded the NCFLBC in triumph in June 1937.[16] This decision also suspended efforts to pressure individual states to rewrite their obscenity codes in light of the *U.S. vs. One Package* decision; thus, in most states contraception remained classed as obscene.[17]

One argument for halting legislative efforts was that prosecution was so rare. As early as 1929, the ABCL began arguing that the shift in public opinion had already made the Comstock Act a dead law. And public opinion was behind the activists. By 1938, a survey conducted by the *Ladies Home Journal* found that 79 percent of women approved of birth control, and of those who disapproved, less than 1 percent gave its legal status as the reason.[18] The ABCL believed that resources spent trying to change the law would be better spent founding clinics and state organizations.[19] Most clinics, even Sanger's BCCRB, operated on this assumption, regularly violating the law by mailing brochures, sending progress reports to the ABCL, announcing fund-raising dinners in local newspapers, and ordering supplies from mail-order houses. Some among them skirted the law on a grand scale. Sanger needed thousands of diaphragms to treat the BCCRB's patients. In the 1920s she smuggled them into the United States from Germany, via the Canadian office of her husband's Three-in-One Oil Company, where they were repackaged in unmarked boxes and forwarded to New York.[20] In Cleveland, activists got around the prohibition by having Morris Black, a garment manufacturer whose wife, Lenore, was a member of the CMHA, carry diaphragms and condoms from New York in extra suitcases on his business trips.[21] We lack the details on how most clinics obtained their supplies, but most had to have broken the law by ordering devices and preparations from companies like Holland-Rantos (New York) and the Clinic Supply Company (Chicago), firms that formed part of a burgeoning American contraceptive industry in the 1930s. To avoid prosecution, these businesses advertised the materials as "feminine hygiene" products, only suggesting a contraceptive function.[22]

Often legal challenges to the clinic's work came *before* the clinic opened, not once it was established. In Chicago, efforts to found a clinic in 1923 were blocked by the city's commissioner of health, who refused the Illinois Birth Control League's application for a license on the grounds that contraception was detrimental to public welfare. The IBCL took the city to court and eventually won a judicial ruling that enabled them to open.[23] Prosecution was uneven, and often subject to the whim or aggressiveness of local district attorneys and other politicians, as well as pressure from opponents of birth control. While activists relied on the nullification argument, they could not guarantee that their clinics would operate safely should a district attorney suddenly begin to enforce the law as written. In Connecticut, the district attorney in Bridgeport refused to prosecute a newly formed clinic, but in Waterbury, authorities raided and closed the local hospital clinic. In Milwaukee, a fledgling clinic ran afoul of the district attorney's office, but the problems were resolved and the clinic was allowed to remain open. Several years later, with a new district attorney in office, the clinic was infiltrated, raided, and prosecuted.[24]

This uncertainty might have created a tense atmosphere of expected arrests and closings. But after the first few years of a clinic's existence, staff stopped worrying. After all, the activists were among the social pillars of their communities. Prosecuting them for obscenity would require more bravery than they believed law enforcement could muster. Activists believed that the courts would prosecute clinics who used lay staff to distribute information, but look the other way if advice was provided by a physician. As BCLM president Linda Hawkridge said after her arrest in Massachusetts, "We have nothing to hide. We have never denied that we gave contraceptive advice, for we consider that a doctor has the right to do what he can to preserve the life of his patients."[25] Activists doubted that police would arrest doctors, and certainly did not believe they could be convicted when treating a woman with a medical reason to practice contraception.

Clinic activists were right about the prosecutors. Of the 650 clinics operating in the United States between 1916 and 1940, I have found only sixteen raids. But of those sixteen clinics, fourteen were shut down, one remained open, and one closed voluntarily shortly afterwards.[26] The BCCRB was the only one to survive its 1929 police raid. The charges were dropped after physicians and the general public protested.[27] When the police raided Sanger's first clinic in 1916, they were more successful. Sanger and her sister Ethel Byrne were convicted and imprisoned, each sentenced to thirty days in the workhouse.[28]

In later clinic prosecutions, the social status of the activists served to mitigate against such punishments. Even when convicted, clinic activists in the 1930s were fined and in most cases never spent a night in prison.

In 1937 and 1939, a flurry of state prosecutions in Massachusetts and Connecticut demonstrated that despite the *One Package* ruling and in the teeth of the nullification argument, a determined state could easily close down clinics. In June of 1937 the Birth Control League of Massachusetts's four clinics were raided and league officers arrested. Convicted, they were fined and forced to close all six of their clinics pending a 1938 appeal. Despite the setback, the activists were confident of victory, believing as Hannah Stone remarked, "All the Massachusetts police can accomplish by closing birth control clinics is to prevent for a time the poor and indigent women from obtaining information that wealthier women can obtain from their private physicians. It is inconceivable that the higher court will uphold the decision of the Salem and Brookline judges. The day of witch hunting has passed. It is no more possible to stem the flow of contraceptive knowledge than to stem the tides of the ocean that wash the shores of Massachusetts."[29]

But Stone and the other activists were wrong. The Massachusetts appeal was denied, and clinics in that state closed permanently. Shortly after the Massachusetts decision, Connecticut, which had the most stringent anti-contraceptive laws in the nation, followed suit. After years of ignoring its illicit clinics, police raided the Waterbury Hospital clinic in 1939, arresting the three physicians in charge. The Waterbury case is particularly interesting because it was a hospital clinic, and activists had long argued that such clinics were viewed as more respectable than those operated by lay women. In both Massachusetts and Connecticut, the impetus for the raids came from the local Catholic Church, whose priests publicly attacked the clinics and demanded their closure.[30] Contraceptive devices were seized and subpoenas issued for clinic records, and a week later the physicians in charge were arrested for aiding and abetting violations of the state law that banned the use of contraceptives. Though the clinic reformers won the first case in September 1939, they lost on appeal in 1940. All Connecticut clinics were closed down and it would be twenty years before they reopened.[31]

The Connecticut and Massachusetts birth control activists were caught unprepared. Upon advice from the ABCL, they pursued a strategy of quiet negotiation, basing their defense on the physician's right to determine the best treatment for patients. Sanger felt the prosecutions were part of an "insidious campaign" to shut down birth control efforts, but 1940 did not usher in a decade of setbacks for birth control clinics. Against the anomalies of Connecticut and Massachusetts, the nullification theory held. Birth control was winning the public relations battle; in 1940, Gallup reported that 72 percent of Americans believed the government should offer birth control to any married person who wanted it, and for those under thirty, the figure rose to 80 percent.[32]

But in another way, the Comstock Laws did restrict the birth control movement's ability to push national plans and programs. Though the federal Comstock Act affected all states due to its restrictions on the mail, each state passed its own obscenity statute, often called "little Comstock laws," to define the nature of obscene material.[33] In most cases, birth control was included in some form, and with its legal status different in each state, efforts to develop a cohesive national policy for clinics was difficult. When Sanger toured the nation exhorting activists to open clinics like the BCCRB, those inspired to follow sometimes took years to determine whether doing so was legal in their state and whether they could risk violating local laws.[34] The legal question led some to shy from opening clinics, focusing instead on legislative or educational programs.

The variety in state laws also hampered the creation of nationwide clinic standards. New York State's laws had an inordinate impact on the creation of standards, as it was the home base of both Sanger and the ABCL. In that state, there had to be a medical reason for prescribing birth control, and this led to a more medicalized movement, focusing on clinics, cooperation with physicians, and health-based arguments for contraception.[35] As the largest and most widely publicized clinic in the nation, Sanger's BCCRB offered other clinics guidance on clinical practice and contraceptive research. Compared to the legal situation in other states, New York's laws were restrictive, and had Sanger based the movement in a more lenient state, clinics might have developed very differently. One might ask, given New York's limitations, why Sanger centered the movement there, when she could have opened less-medicalized clinics almost anywhere else. She did consider opening clinics in Chicago in 1917, but New York was her home and the home of her wealthy donors. By 1923, Sanger was convinced that she needed to work with—not against—the medical profession, and while she interpreted the state's restrictions broadly, she believed that access to birth control should be handled by doctors as preventive medicine.[36]

The inability of birth control activists to repeal the Comstock Act at the federal level or to succeed in efforts to repeal state laws hampered efforts to establish clinics in hospitals and settlement houses. Until 1970, birth control was still technically obscene. Though rarely prosecuted, the Comstock Act provided an easy reason to ignore birth control. Prosecutions, rare though they were, underscored the questionable legal basis upon which most clinic operations rested, threatening the chances of state-supported birth control.

Clinics and Public Health

Activists believed that every woman had the right to contraceptives and that the state should provide birth control for a woman who could not afford it. For Sanger, birth control's benefits to the woman, the family, the community, and the state outweighed the expense and any objections. Among the tactics used to attract government interest and support, the most compelling was the argument that access to birth control could lower infant and maternal mortality rates. This was an area of government concern, and activists offered another weapon with which to address the problem. The situation was serious—in 1916, approximately 100 infants of every 1,000 born died before reaching their first birthday, an estimated 300,000 annually. Maternal mortality was also high, an appalling 91 per 10,000 in 1918, over twice the rate of other industrialized nations.[37] Activists believed that birth control could attract middle-class and government support by focusing on its ability to save the lives of mothers and children, rather than on its impact on women's liberation and sexual autonomy.

Infant mortality, defined as the deaths of children before they reached their first birthday, was caused by prematurity, congenital defects, and birth injuries, all difficult to cure or even prevent; but infant mortality was also affected by socioeconomic and environmental problems. Gastrointestinal disease, tuberculosis, and malnutrition were linked to the family's income levels and ability to secure decent housing. Maternal mortality, caused by postnatal complications such as sepsis, toxaemia, or hemorrhage, was often linked to botched abortions. As with infant mortality, socioeconomic factors, such as the availability of prenatal care, the expertise of doctors or midwives, and the cleanliness of the environment, were crucial factors in reducing rates.[38]

Efforts to reduce mortality rates for women and children took many forms; some were designed to eliminate one factor while others aimed more broadly. The pure-milk campaign, which began in the 1870s, for example, sought to reduce infant deaths from gastrointestinal ailments contracted from tainted milk. Milk stations educated urban working-class women about the need for pure milk, and made it available at reduced costs. To reduce maternal deaths from sepsis, activists campaigned to license or do away with midwives, blaming them for improper hygiene. More general efforts included widows' pensions to provide food and shelter for dependent children, visiting nurse programs, and prenatal clinics that screened working-class women and their children for signs of trouble. Educational efforts to teach working-class women hygienic methods of housework or nutrition made homes less susceptible to contagion.[39]

As a tool for public health, birth control improved the working-class family's overall environment, rather than targeting any one cause of mortality. It might not save any one specific infant or mother, but birth control generally raised the standard of living. Women who practiced birth control were less likely to die of complications from childbirth and their children were more likely to survive their first year. Infant mortality rates were lower in smaller families, especially where there was an interval of two or more years between births. Smaller families were associated with the middle class, but activists argued that smaller family size benefited the poor as well. Activists also believed that birth control could reduce maternal mortality by reducing the numbers of women who sought abortions. They backed up this contention with statistics, revealing that many patients used abortion as a method of birth control before attending the clinic. They argued that repeated childbearing debilitated women, making them easier prey to disease and complications of childbirth. Thus, birth control enabled a closer connection between a family's environment (both health and economic) and its size, reducing death rates and eventually contributing to population growth, as more children survived to adulthood and their mothers lived longer lives.[40]

Despite the specter of infant and maternal mortality, the federal government was reluctant to provide direct relief to the poor. Its agencies, the Children's Bureau and U.S. Public Health Service, were restricted to education and data gathering, with no mandate to ensure American health through medical care.[41] The medical profession opposed state-sponsored medicine and many social workers railed against handouts of any kind, associating them with moral weakness, poverty, and disease. Educational efforts offered the government a way to address the problem without offending these powerful partners or challenging the idea that poverty could be escaped through personal betterment efforts.[42]

Individual doctors could and often did support birth control when confronted by a worried patient requesting aid, most making such decisions in private. Shrouded in doctor-patient confidentiality, many doctors believed that they could tell when a patient truly needed help and when she sought birth control for selfish or immoral reasons. These doctors seemed more comfortable prescribing contraceptives or referring patients to clinics than they were publicly supporting patients' rights to contraceptive information. When dealing with a particular case, doctors easily set aside concerns over socialized medicine or morality because they could see the social, eugenic, or medical reason why the patient needed the information. Thus, individual doctors might support the movement by working in clinics or by advising their patients about contraception, but when they organized in groups and societies, support often dried up. Medical organizations were created to defend the rights of physicians and maintain standards of quality in the profession. In looking out for the needs of doctors as a group, medical societies tended to oppose any provision of medical services by lay people or the government. They stymied efforts to create national health insurance. These threats to their livelihood and their medical monopoly occupied state, local, and national medical societies throughout this period.[43] Also, just as they were able to do in social-work groups and political parties, Catholic physicians blocked birth control endorsements. Catholic doctors generally refused their patients any information on contraception, if anecdotes from patient letters can be believed. Other physicians, such as specialists in tuberculosis and venereal disease, for example, were more likely to support birth control clinics because they saw the damaging effects of repeated pregnancies.

The Children's Bureau, which headed the government's response to infant and maternal mortality until the mid-1930s, was a fact-finding organization responsible for many other issues, including child labor, juvenile delinquency, illegitimacy, and mothers' pensions. Barred by its charter from giving direct aid or medical care, the CB instead issued advisory bulletins, campaigned for the extension of birth registration and data collection to all states, researched the causes and extent of infant and maternal mortality, and oversaw programs carried out by state and local government agencies. Children's Bureau studies proved the relationship between poverty and infant mortality, demonstrating that most deaths could be prevented with good prenatal care.[44] But the CB lacked clout in Washington. Its lay female staff faced opposition from the male-dominated Public Health Service as well as the American Medical Association (AMA), both of which opposed state-subsidized medicine. Some women's groups also questioned the right of unmarried women "experts" to tell married mothers how to raise their children. As this opposition increased, the CB tried to keep a low profile, backing away from controversial issues such as birth control, and instead focusing closely on children's needs, even to the detriment of women's needs.[45]

The highpoint of the CB's efforts to reduce maternal and infant mortality was the passage of the 1921 Sheppard-Towner Maternity and Infant Protection Act, which provided federal matching funds for state programs that used visiting nurses, clinics, and instruction to reduce infant and maternal mortality. Supported by many women's groups, the bill passed in the early days of women's suffrage, when legislators feared that women might vote as a block. Careful to placate medical societies, the CB limited the Sheppard-Towner clinics to treat only women and ruled that any sick children that were brought to the clinic had to be referred to a private physician.[46]

Activists tried to use Sheppard-Towner legislation to secure federal and state funding for birth control clinics. Both Sanger and Mary Ware Dennett lobbied the CB to allow government-funded infant and maternal health clinics to include contraceptive advice, but the CB, already under fire for involving itself in medical work, flatly refused to consider it. Instead, the CB took "no stand" on the issue of birth control, denying accusations that the clinics would offer contraceptive advice. Though the CB received thousands of letters each year asking for birth control help, they refused to provide any information and would not even pass the letters to birth control activists who wanted to answer them. The CB's tactics with regard to birth control defended the agency's gains but also revealed that its values on sex and motherhood were those of older, more conservative women. The social workers at the CB directed their efforts and propaganda toward the more palatable mission of saving children, not preventing them from being born. Perhaps they feared the taint of feminism, but more likely they believed that motherhood was the natural function of most women (though not themselves). Supporting efforts to help women avoid motherhood did not appeal to their world views.[47]

The Sheppard-Towner experiment was short-lived and limited in scope. It was underfunded ($1.4 million for 1922 and $1.2 million per year from 1923 to 1929). Its staff could not enter prospective patients' homes without being invited, nor could they offer any kind of medical advice. Despite these shortcomings, Sheppard-Towner programs were begun in all but three states, and infant mortality rates declined by 11 percent overall and by 47 percent from the gastrointestinal diseases that were most easily addressed through educational programs. Maternal mortality did not decline.[48] The CB estimated that in the seven years that the program was in action, sixty thousand babies had been saved.[49]

Despite promising results, the CB was unable to defend and protect the program, and efforts to reauthorize the bill in Congress failed. The Sheppard-Towner Act expired in 1929.[50] This failure, largely at the hands of the medical profession, was based on virulent opposition to "socialized medicine" as well as to efforts by lay women to "dabble in medicine," refrains that equally applied to birth control clinics. But more than that, it reflected the medical profession's redefinition of its role with its patients. After the Sheppard-Towner program underscored the importance of preventive health, checkups and regular physical examinations became part of a physician's private practice. Once the program ended, efforts to reintroduce similar legislation failed.[51] The legacy of the Sheppard-Towner program was felt most strongly at the local level. The program stimulated interest in preventive care and in the state's role in public health. Though most programs were abandoned once the federal subsidies ran out, work continued in sixteen states, albeit at a reduced level. North Carolina was one of those states, appropriating funds in the early 1930s for maternal and child health care that expanded with the availability of Social Security funds.[52]

In 1929, President Hoover put the PHS in charge of infant and maternal health programs, despite the agency's lack of interest. Having opposed the creation of the CB and its involvement in infant and maternal welfare programs, the PHS focused its efforts on eradicating contagious diseases, especially venereal disease. They saw themselves as "scientific," in contrast to the CB, which one PHS officer described as "a group of sentimental women . . . interested solely in the welfare of mothers and infants." If the CB had its constituents, so did the PHS. Made up of physicians, the PHS was staunch in its defense of private practice. Along with the AMA, the PHS fought plans to federally fund public health, arguing that direct medical care remained the responsibility of private practitioners, not the government.[53] With this mind-set, it is not surprising that the PHS did little to relieve infant and maternal mortality until the mid-1930s.

The onset of the Great Depression increased demands on government in all aspects of social policy. In response, New Dealers offered new government programs that provided direct aid. The Social Security Act of 1935 (SSA) offered the nation's first comprehensive welfare program, comprising old age benefits, unemployment, and worker's compensation. It drew the line at offering direct medical care or universal health insurance due to opposition from the medical profession and the cost of such programs. However, Title V of the SSA reinstated maternal and child welfare services, overseen jointly by the CB and PHS, once more providing federal grants to states. Unlike in the 1920s, Catholic lobbyists made certain that the program could not include contraceptives.[54] The SSA's Title VI enlarged the PHS's role, enabling it to provide grants to create state and local health departments. Under a new surgeon general, Thomas S. Parran, the PHS accepted the challenge of jump-starting state health departments, laboring in a failed effort to secure national health insurance, a rare instance where the agency worked against organized medicine's wishes.[55]

When birth control was included in public health programs, it was rarely in the form of a brick-and-mortar clinic. Instead, states established visiting nurse programs to reach the rural poor. They advised patients on a wide variety of health concerns, including contraception, but avoided the kind of explicit government support for contraception that an actual clinic would signal.[56] With the availability of government funding under the Social Security Act in 1935, more state and local health departments were created, most focusing on combating venereal disease, tuberculosis, mental illness, industrial dangers, and poor dental health. Relying on what they knew best, the PHS set up programs under the SSA that targeted specific population groups, a tactic that Congress preferred to more general programs.[57]

In 1938–39, national birth control organizations tried once more to pressure the PHS and CB to support birth control. The BCCRB harnessed public support in a targeted letter-writing campaign aimed at Surgeon General Thomas Parran and CB head Katharine Lenroot and seeking explicit inclusion of contraception in Social Security–funded programs. They orchestrated mailing campaigns to state health departments, hoping to secure support from these agencies. Parran rejected the demands, claiming that birth control should "be considered by individual physicians in dealing with patients," and noting that there were "larger issues of population which need much further scientific study before I feel we are in a position to consider widespread administrative action through public health agencies." Katharine Lenroot refused to even discuss it, repeating the CB's "consistent policy . . . to take no position with reference to birth control." Ellen Chesler argues that Lenroot feared birth control's potential role in population decline and economic stagnation, and also believed that childbearing should not be a privilege of wealth. Both the PHS and the CB eased their opposition in the 1940s, but it was not until the 1960s that family planning became an integral part of government health provision.[58]

The ABCL tried low-key lobbying at state health departments to subsidize contraceptive clinics, believing that local birth control activists would have the best chance of success. The ABCL drafted propaganda material specifically for public health centers and for publication in *Health Officer*, the PHS's journal. After 1937, the ABCL convinced the PHS to pass inquiries they received on birth control to the league. The ABCL also announced in its clinic guidelines that the era of lay birth control clinics was drawing to a close, superseded by doctor-controlled clinics in state health departments.[59] It was surely premature, for only 11 percent of almost five hundred clinics were operated by state governments. In 1938, the ABCL acknowledged as much when it created guidelines for health department clinics, asserting the need to use physicians, rather than public health nurses, as supervisors. In cases where an independent clinic was already in operation, the ABCL now suggested that rather than start a new clinic, a health department ought to refer patients to the existing clinic and subsidize the costs. This would ensure that the patient received expert treatment and that detailed records would be maintained.[60]

By the end of the 1930s, neither Sanger nor the BCFA was able to secure significant federal support or funding for birth control. As late as May 1939, Sanger confided to a friend that they were still unsure whether "government officials are actually forbidden to promote birth control—or whether this statement is used as a cloak to shield those responsible for leadership from taking an active role." Though Sanger argued that the government could not "ignore the will of the people" forever, the pace of change was glacial.[61]

Agitation for public-health-based birth control clinics was always more successful at the local level than on the national stage. The social prestige of local birth control activists, combined with efforts to reduce infant and maternal mortality, convinced some local public health officers to participate, either by aiding local clinics or providing services in their own centers. But government-sponsored and supported clinics remained rare and ephemeral in the interwar period, despite the efforts of activists to encourage them.

SEVEN

Local Clinics and National Organizations

Most historians of the birth control movement have focused on the extremes: either investigating the national movement and its leaders or detailing the history of a specific league or clinic. This has led to two divergent interpretations. National studies assume that organizations like the ABCL or BCCRB were models for local leagues and clinics and controlled clinic policy and staff from their New York City offices.[1] Each of the local studies argues against that narrative, pronouncing their clinic or league an anomaly, a maverick that did not fit the mold. As these histories multiply, it is time to rethink the mold.[2]

The national leagues operating in the 1920s and 1930s were the ABCL, the NCFLBC, and the BCFA. Each of these organizations purported to represent the entire country and worked to popularize birth control. The ABCL and BCFA were based in New York City, while the NCFLBC had offices in New York, Washington, D.C., and briefly in Los Angeles. The ABCL was organized into state and city affiliates. The BCFA operated similarly, but added a layer of regional directors to advise and oversee state leagues. But neither organization had true national coverage. By the mid-1930s, the ABCL only had organized in twenty-one of the forty-eight states; by 1939, the BCFA only had organizations in twenty-nine.[3] The NCFLBC, chiefly a lobbying organization, did better, having set up thirty-seven state chairmen and an additional ninety-seven congressional district chairs to marshal support in key areas.[4] They also established four regional chairmanships, tasked to expand work into unorganized regions.

All three groups aimed to organize the whole nation and gathered, processed, and reported information on birth control's progress to its members and the public. The ABCL and BCFA issued a monthly journal, the *BCR*, and the NCFLBC sent circular letters and short newsletters reporting their activities and asking for specific cooperation. All three served as clearinghouses for information on contraceptive methods, laws, practices, and justifications and provided expert advice and support for anyone seeking to join the movement. Their efforts to organize states and territories often led to the expansion of clinics and leagues, as field workers and organizers traveled around the country to stir up activity.[5]

The BCCRB has not traditionally been seen as a national birth control organization, but I would argue that in the 1930s it was the most important organization for clinic activists.[6] The BCCRB was more than just a clinic. While its first priority was to treat patients, it did not stop there. It tested and reported the effectiveness of a range of contraceptives, analyzed and reported on patients' experiences, created instructional literature, gave lectures, organized conferences, and offered educational services on contraception for doctors and nurses. Once Sanger split from the ABCL in 1929, the BCCRB became her chief vehicle for providing practical advice. At one time or another, the BCCRB was affiliated with all three national organizations and overlapped with their work. Especially after Sanger founded the NCFLBC in 1929, letters written to one organization might be answered by the other. Sometimes staff held positions in both organizations, further confusing any distinctions between them.[7]

Even when we examine its primary function—patient care—the BCCRB was an anomaly. It treated many more patients than its nearest competitor, more in a year than many clinics did in a decade. Sanger promoted the BCCRB heavily, making it the touchstone for anyone seeking instruction on birth control methods, research, or clinical services. While other important clinics and leagues, like those run by the IBCL and CMHA, were occasionally asked for advice, the requests coming to Sanger and the BCCRB were constant.

With four organizations on the national scene, local activists had plenty of opportunities to work with skilled and experienced activists. They had models to follow, data to analyze, and ready assistance when they ran into trouble.

Rather than focus solely on the activities of the national organizations or local activists, let us look at how these groups interacted. Leagues and clinics were not usually organized at the behest of a central office, nor did they spread systematically throughout regions or states. Anyone could organize a clinic in any city without the permission of the local, county, state, or national birth control league. There was no requirement that birth control clinics affiliate with either the ABCL or the BCCRB, and there were no repercussions if their policies and practices diverged from those drafted by national organizations.

One source of the confusion about the role of the national organization comes from the ABCL. They worked to create a hierarchical movement that clearly divided tasks and responsibility to different groups. At the national level, the ABCL would be responsible for the overall direction of the movement, the educational and public relations aspects of it, and the organizing of state leagues. State leagues would report on their work to the national movement, help city leagues, and foster the spread of birth control in their state by organizing new city groups. City leagues organized clinics in their towns, dealt with local leaders, and reported on their progress to the state leagues. Their plan was extremely organized and regimented, but unfortunately, it was mostly wishful thinking. In practice, many clinics operated without the supervision of a city-based birth control league or without any close connection to the state or national leagues. Cities organized flourishing leagues without state organizations to guide and direct them. Some clinics worked directly with national leaders, while others shunned the national movement altogether. It was not the structured, organized movement the ABCL wanted to see. Instead the spread of clinics and leagues crossed the nation like a spider web, linked loosely together, with activity in some places outpacing others. It was a fragile movement, with weak and easily broken links. National leaders looked out upon the entire web, promoting it as a big idea, but any effort to direct its development risked breaking the loose strands that held everything together.

The Clinic's Life Cycle

Birth control clinics were born, nurtured, and either took flight, generating enough support and acceptance to continue to operate each year, or they crashed, closing after running afoul of opposition, a lack of financial support, or a lack of interest. The national birth control movement was intimately concerned with the start of this life cycle, encouraging the founding of clinics, but had less influence over whether an individual clinic would stand or fall.

At the start of their work, clinic activists relied most heavily on the national movement, in particular, on Margaret Sanger.[8] Activists read about her in the newspapers, discussed her books and articles, flocked to her lectures, and, most importantly, heeded her exhortations to form birth control clinics and leagues. Even those who opposed her work, such as the physicians of the CMH, were inspired to build hospital and public health clinics as an alternative to her model. Sanger's greatest influence was on lay women. Before her campaign began, the only role they had in the birth control movement was as consumers. In order to create an active and vital movement, Sanger tapped networks of wealthy and committed women seeking important causes and she gave them a stirring social welfare rationale for birth control that inspired them to take on the work.

This inspiration was the most important aid the national birth control movement provided to local activists, but it did not always lead immediately to the founding of a clinic. As individual women heard of the movement, some tried to interest friends, but these efforts were often muted. It could be difficult to learn that a group was forming, as one Chicago Woman's Club member recalled: "I heard murmuring, around the edges, of meetings behind closed doors." Even as late as 1931, Margaret Cohen of the Buffalo Family Relations Clinic described a furtive beginning: "All our plans had to be made in secret. Birth Control was definitely something you didn't discuss in the 1930s, except behind closed doors. Not only were the doors closed on the first meeting . . . they were locked from inside. We didn't want anyone peeking in."[9]

Once they committed to forming a birth control clinic, while many local activists sought guidance from Sanger and her New York associates, others were perfectly capable of creating their own vision of a birth control clinic. Clinics run by the CMHA, the Cincinnati Committee for Maternal Health, and even the IBCL, developed differently according to the strengths of local organizers, public perceptions of birth control, and the relative power of organized medicine in each city. In some cases, leagues decided to work for birth control education or lobbying, but did not want to open a clinic. Some doctors were inspired to help the women in their cities, occasionally opening private clinics to offer reduced-price services for poor women. Few of these groups and individuals would have conceived of doing such work without the publicity Sanger garnered for birth control.[10]

From 1916 through the prosperous 1920s, the stock market crash, and the ensuing Depression, Sanger inspired followers using a mix of old and new rationales to urge ever-increasing numbers of men and women to participate in the birth control movement. But she was not alone. The ABCL sent other workers into the field to help organize leagues and drum up support. Executive Secretary Anne Kennedy spoke to social work and women's organizations, while Medical Director James F. Cooper addressed medical men. Clinicians like Hannah Stone often spoke to groups in the New York metropolitan area, and in the 1930s the ABCL, NCFLBC, and BCCRB field workers and organizers, like Doris Davidson, Ruth Smith, Marion Post, Joyce Ely, and James Toy, traveled the country, helping launch local leagues and clinics across the nation.[11]

The first public lecture on birth control in a city often predated the creation of the local league or clinic. A small group interested in the topic would usually contact Sanger or the ABCL to arrange an event. In some cases, ABCL secretaries would write women's clubs in cities along train routes when Sanger was on a cross-country tour, trying to find a venue for her to speak. These splashy mass meetings garnered headlines in the local papers for days in advance and full coverage of the speech and its sponsors.[12] Sanger's goal was to leave the city with a nucleus of local activists inspired to organize a league, and eventually a clinic. She knew how to secure publicity, to pitch the need for birth control in terms that would appeal to society women, doctors, and social workers, and she promised the assistance of her national organization to the fledgling league. She might appear at several venues in a particular city, often held on the same day, one sponsored by the local woman's club, one by a social service agency, and another by the medical society. Sanger tailored her speeches to her expected audiences. To a woman's club she might stress the many benefits birth control offered for the health of women and children. To social workers, she would emphasize the economic benefits that welfare families would reap if they had fewer mouths to feed. For doctors, it was the clinical nature of the work she highlighted, stressing that they wanted to work *with* physicians, not *against* them. She claimed that birth control could reduce the risks of pregnancy for women suffering from conditions like heart and kidney disease. In the 1930s, her arguments shifted to address the needs of a struggling social welfare system, focused on amending restrictive and outdated federal and state laws, helping reduce the welfare burden by limiting family size, and calling for government-supported birth control clinics as an essential public health measure.[13]

These public events helped interest coalesce into action, even though it was not always immediate. Instructed to "canvass every wealthy woman and every active woman volunteer in charity," organizers tried to identify women willing to at least listen to the need for a clinic. Luncheon meetings were held to attract women who "represented both millions in money and also nearly every philanthropy in town," and efforts were made to identify "a local leader in the medical profession," someone "perhaps secretly, quite sympathetic and humanely concerned about the poverty-stricken mothers-of-many who need contraception in his town."[14]

Detroit offers an example. Emma Goldman first spoke there in November 1915. Sanger followed in May 1916, encouraging an early organizational effort that petered out in 1918. In 1921, Mrs. William McGraw attended the ABCL's inaugural New York conference in November 1921 and formed a Detroit committee in January 1922. McGraw asked Sanger to come and speak in February of 1922, an event that jump-started the Detroit Birth Control League. It took five more years of organizing before they were able to open the Detroit Mother's Clinic in 1927. Of McGraw's early efforts, her daughter recalled, "Many of my mother's friends begged her not to take part in the work. One very prominent doctor told her that she was making a serious mistake. This same physician was happy to sit at the speaker's table at a later luncheon meeting."[15]

While mass meetings were spectacular events, the smaller, private meetings arranged for Sanger and other field workers were often equally important. There they met with women, doctors, nurses, and social workers in less formal settings, at teas and luncheons in private homes. In these drawing rooms, local activists could ask practical questions, introduce Sanger to key individuals whose support they needed, and figure out the best way to get a clinic off the ground. Time after time, as happened in Buffalo in 1932, after gathering the various medical and lay interests in the city in one room, Sanger promised, "There will be a clinic in Buffalo in a very short time."[16]

New Jersey offers an example of the kind of sustained effort that could be made to get the movement started in a region. Finding their neighboring state "asleep as far as Birth Control was concerned," the ABCL sent field worker Henrietta Hart around the state from January to March 1927. Hart helped set up local committees in seven communities. In April, Hannah Stone addressed a general meeting of these committees, advising them on clinic procedures, and this meeting resulted in the creation of the New Jersey Birth Control League. James Cooper followed in June, meeting with medical men. At the end of the month, Sanger met the heads of the committees, an event described as "an inspirational occasion." New Jersey leader Kate Belcher acknowledged their debt to the ABCL: "To awaken a state first to the necessity and second to the moral and financial responsibility of conducting a Birth Control clinic in face of prejudice, ignorance and *fear of legal consequences* is no small task. Far from considering the goal as reached or finished when the Clinic will be opened, the League appreciates that its real work is just beginning. But with the inspiration of our great leader Margaret Sanger and the cooperation of the National organization, we hope we can accomplish this."[17]

This focused work on one state was not the norm and was no doubt facilitated by New Jersey's proximity to New York, but it shows how national leaders could go after a region using all its resources to build birth control activities where there were none. In most cases, the impetus for a Sanger visit came from the local activists. Sanger and the ABCL received requests from all over the country, far more than they could accommodate each year.[18]

Clinic activists sought advice from the national movement on how to operate a clinic. Asked the same questions over and over, Sanger, the ABCL, and the BCCRB began to codify the answers, first in the forms of letters, and later in pamphlets and articles. The ABCL and BCCRB created printed brochures and other literature, sample patient cards, and reports on various brands of contraceptives. Sanger, in particular, was known to invite clinic doctors and staff to come to New York and "spend any amount of time" at the BCCRB until they felt comfortable returning home and starting their own service.[19]

Once the clinics were operational, their interactions with the national movement changed. They did not need inspiration any longer; they needed practical assistance: money, supplies, and the participation of activists and patients. Here the national movement was of less use. Chronically short-funded, even before Sanger split from it, the ABCL sought funds from its affiliates; it did not have the resources to support clinics or supply them with contraceptives. Nor could the national movement ensure that local physicians would be willing to staff a clinic. It was even less likely that they would be able to offer substantial help attracting patients, especially given the Comstock Act's bans on mailed information. Despite the national movement's help in birthing the clinic, once it was functioning, local activists were expected to keep it going.

National organizations continued to provide some aid. The *BCR* and other journals and form letters kept local activists apprised of what was going on, not only in the United States but around the world. The BCR published articles written by various clinic activists about their work, and also included a geographically arranged "News Notes" at the back of each issue that described the doings of clinics and leagues, reported on speeches, and noted prominent legal cases. The *JOC*, first published in 1935, was even more focused on clinic work, publishing annual reports, descriptions of specific clinics, and articles about methods and clinical practice.

Leagues still beseeched Sanger to travel to their cities, even after the clinics were opened. They hoped that she would bring them more attention, headlines, and donations if she would launch their funding drives or attend their annual meetings. As the requests grew more frequent and farther afield, Sanger could not accommodate all of them. But activists persisted in inviting her year after year. If they were able to secure Sanger's participation, many organizations did what the Indianapolis Maternal Health League did; they immediately went on a large-scale funding drive, capped by a tea where Sanger addressed twelve hundred people, holding them in "rapt attention."[20]

Regardless of the assistance that the national movement provided, I have not come across a single case where a national organization or leader was able to keep an ailing clinic alive or overcome attempts to prosecute and close a clinic. There were real limits to the ability of any outside organization to affect local practices.

The Vast Network of Clinics

Clinics were one yardstick that the national movement used to measure its progress. How many states had they organized? How many cities possessed clinics, and how many patients were seen each year? When these figures were increasing, the movement was healthy and strong; if they began declining, activists tried to understand what was going wrong. Without affiliates and clinics dotting the map, the national organizations ran the risk of becoming what Sanger derided as "paper organizations," ones that existed only on letterhead, with no connection to the grassroots activists. Up until the mid-1930s, in order to keep expanding and showing progress, national activists put most of their resources into founding new clinics and organizing new territories; they were far less interested in what actually happened at each clinic.

National organizations gathered information about each clinic in the country, using that information to compile clinic directories that were produced several times a year.[21] These were listings by state and city of every clinic of which the national movement was aware. As the 1930s progressed, leagues sought additional information from the clinics, sometimes sending out forms for them to record annual patient data, or requesting a copy of the clinic's annual report. With this information, the ABCL, BCCRB, or BCFA advised those patients, activists, or physicians who contacted them with information about the closest clinic to them and its staff.

In the 1930s, the proliferation of national organizations and activists, including the ABCL, Sanger, the BCCRB, and the NCFLBC, competed more fiercely for the attention and participation of grassroots organizations and local activists. An unwritten agreement had been made that assigned the ABCL responsibility for organizing leagues, the NCFLBC for lobbying, and the BCCRB for contraceptive research and direct aid to clinics. Even if the organizations had intended to stick to these spheres, it would have been difficult, as they were so interconnected. But with relations between the leagues acrimonious, none of them honored the agreement. An NCFLBC state organizer might visit a city to publicize the current birth control bill and secure endorsements to take to Congress, but when asked advice on forming a league or clinic group, she would happily offer aid. The ABCL organizers, supposed to be creating new leagues, had no compunction about offering advice on clinic creation, methods, and operations. And the BCCRB's organizers were eager to advise interested women on starting a league and then a clinic, suggesting that they not bother with the ABCL. Workers in the field pretty much helped local activists create whatever sort of organization they wanted, and rarely mentioned the other groups.[22]

In the early 1930s, the ABCL began trying to implement its vision of a hierarchical movement. Their field workers started out trying to organize state leagues where there were none, in the hopes that those leagues would then canvass the state for birth control. The ABCL saw this approach as more efficient, allowing them to intensively organize in one state or region to speed results. In the spring of 1933, for example, the ABCL sent field worker Clara Louise McGraw to the South, where birth control work was not well organized. In Virginia and Georgia she created state birth control organizations, from scratch in Virginia, and by cajoling the existing Atlanta league to take over the entire state. In Kentucky, she helped the state league secure a medical advisory board. In an extended visit lasting several months, she traveled to seven states, meeting a wide variety of individuals and organizations. Marion Post, dispatched to Illinois for five weeks in 1937, helped the

IBCL organize committees in six cities in the central and southern parts of the state. The ABCL's field workers taught local leagues how to expand their reach by setting up satellite organizations, how to organize and cooperate with clinics and leagues that already operated in the state, and how to organize new cities and clinics to spread coverage.[23]

As Sanger directed her attention to federal lobbying in the 1930s, she delegated practical advice work to the BCCRB, including medical director Dr. Hannah Stone and lay field workers. Stone was best suited to provide doctors with specific instruction in prescribing and fitting contraceptives, and was more experienced in day-to-day clinic work than Sanger. Having a physician advise clinicians also helped underscore Sanger's contention that contraception was a medical issue. The BCCRB's executive secretaries advised clinic administrators and board members, and through annual reports, tests of diaphragms and spermicides, and published studies of patient records, offered tangible examples of a successful clinic. The BCCRB continued to work directly with clinics; it did not work through the state leagues.[24]

The NCFLBC, organized by states and congressional districts, used a different tactic to gather grassroots support. They kept up the practice of short visits and public appearances by Sanger and other speakers, but appointed local activists to serve as state chairs. The chairwoman was responsible for securing the endorsements for the bills from individuals and organizations. They then mobilized the supporters, via petition-signing, meetings with congressmen, and fund-raising for the lobbying effort. By co-opting the local activists, the NCFLBC was in constant touch with these local activists. Sometimes the state chairwoman was also the head of the state birth control league, but more often she was not. The NCFLBC worked closely with the BCCRB to provide their members with advice on clinic questions, but also harvested the names and addresses of interested individuals for their lobbying efforts.[25]

In 1935, clinics were expanding at a rapid pace, and national activists began rethinking their relationship with local activists. They recognized that the legitimacy of the lobbying efforts of the ABCL, the BCCRB, and the NCFLBC were linked to the quality of local clinics. To a potential supporter in Dubuque, it did not matter how advanced the BCCRB was in New York City. Her perception of the birth control movement would come chiefly from the reputation of the clinic in her home town. If it was run by physicians of questionable integrity, was shabby or dirty, or if it was rumored to offer abortions, the national movement would be damaged. Poorly implemented birth control jeopardized the movement's ability to attain its major goals—medical acceptance for birth control, legislative reform, and the inclusion of birth control in public health programs. Well-run clinics could positively influence doctors, senators and representatives, and the lay funders the movement needed to continue to grow. Clinic quality became the watchword for the second half of the 1930s.

Clinic activists had always had some standards to strive for, as outlined in the guides published by the national organizations and discussed at birth control conferences. Meeting en masse, birth control activists learned practical clinic administration, ranging from methods of attracting and keeping patients and raising funds to medical procedures and record-keeping.[26] But in the mid-1930s, the idea of general clinic standards morphed into a quality control plan that would certify that individual clinics met the stringent requirements of the national organization. Designed to bring prestige to the local clinic and clout to whichever national organization could claim the most affiliated clinics, these programs were a key factor in the increased competition between Sanger's BCCRB and the ABCL, which finally ended in 1939 with the merger of the two.

The ABCL launched its affiliation program in May 1935 with three aims: to draw unaffiliated clinics and leagues into association with the ABCL; to differentiate between clinics run by affiliated state leagues and those run by independents; and to "discredit the purely commercial clinic." Affiliated clinics had to associate with the ABCL state affiliate (if there was one) and hew to standards that included an ABCL-vetted statement of purpose and admissions policy, a medical board to oversee treatment, the use of approved contraceptive devices, and a financial contribution to the ABCL.[27]

This drive to standardize came from the ABCL's medical committee, headed by Dr. Eric Matsner, who wanted to put clinical practice and contraceptive research more firmly under the control of doctors. The ABCL also hoped to bring social work agencies into the movement as they tried to include birth control in public health programs. It wanted to showcase a more "professional" birth control clinic, one in which work was to be done by paid and trained workers, guided by state leagues and the national activists. The only responsibility that remained for lay volunteers was financing the work.[28]

Most clinics did not adopt the ABCL's standards as written. The league was torn between wanting to make it relatively easy for clinics to affiliate and wanting the standards to mean something. Few clinics were willing to provide financial support to the ABCL, and many institutional clinics were unwilling to join the state birth control organizations. Faced with the possibility of alienating the kinds of clinics they most favored, the ABCL relaxed its standards on a case-by-case basis. It was willing to bend in order to secure cooperation, especially when it realized that many hospital clinics would not affiliate under the initial guidelines. In 1936, the ABCL dropped the requirement that a clinic needed to be part of the state organization.[29] By 1938, it simplified the certification rules further, simplifying data forms and making the certificates, once permanent, now temporary. This required each clinic to reapply every two years, verifying that it still maintained the standards set by the medical committee.[30]

The BCCRB was always interested in clinic development and as early as 1933 had surveyed the nation's clinics, trying to understand how they worked. In 1933, Sanger was already thinking about formalizing the BCCRB's role with other clinics. "I feel that owing to the number of so-called Clinics cropping up like mushrooms all over the country," she instructed Hannah Stone, "that it is time for us, associated with the Clinical Research Bureau, to invite affiliation of such Clinics throughout the country as soon as we know how ethical and sound they are in their technique."[31] Sanger's idea of standardization was different in attitude from that of the ABCL. She wanted to separate clinical work from activism in order to attract broader medical support. She knew through years of association with doctors like Robert Dickinson and S. Adolphus Knopf, that while doctors would accept her, a lay woman, as the leader of the ABCL, or the NCFLBC, they balked at the idea that she controlled the BCCRB. As Knopf put it in 1929: "I fear that you will subject yourself to very severe criticisms because it is generally understood by the medical profession that the head of a medical clinic should be a medically trained man or woman." In the early months of the BCCRB's affiliation campaign, Sanger envisioned creating a new national organization, a "Clinic Association," strictly concerned with matters of contraceptive technique and research. Arguing that the medical profession would not cooperate with birth control groups "while lay people are mixed up in medical projects," Sanger hoped that by organizing the medical and scientific personnel of the clinics, they could get better cooperation from medical organizations, public health workers, and hospital administrators.[32]

The BCCRB's campaign was announced in November 1935, about half a year after the ABCL affiliation program was begun. The BCCRB's affiliations focused on what the national organizations provided to the clinic, not on the requirements the clinic had to meet. The BCCRB offered a fund for clinic startups, providing fifty dollars' worth of contraceptive supplies, sample patient forms, and guidelines for reporting on patient treatment.[33] It conducted a research study of a new cheap contraceptive method, foam powder, inviting certified clinics to join the trial and to receive the experimental product free of charge. The BCCRB only required that the clinic provide feedback on the method.[34] In 1937, the BCCRB started the "Printed Matter Exchange." Each affiliated clinic sent the BCCRB a set of their promotional materials, which the BCCRB then distributed to its other affiliates. Each clinic got a sampling of the materials created by the others and used them as inspiration when revising their publications.[35] The BCCRB published the *JOC* to help link clinicians and clinic administrators and planned a monthly "Clinic Courier" with news and tips for the lay staff. Many of these programs never had a chance to blossom, and were ceased after the merger, but they demonstrated a different kind of affiliation, one of information sharing as opposed to regulation.

The BCCRB and the ABCL had different outlooks on independent clinics. The BCCRB continued to encourage the creation of aggressive, independent clinics, arguing that "clinics financed by public funds are at present much more inaccessible to the average woman seeking advice than the privately organized clinic. . . . In many cases advice is given only when it is likely an additional pregnancy would result in death." The BCCRB advised clinics to accept both indigent and paying patients, and encouraged clinic committees to seek out controversy and publicity, promising that public approval would protect them from prosecution.[36] The BCCRB printed "How to Establish a Birth Control Clinic," which suggested that activists divide responsibility between a lay committee that ran day-to-day operations and raised funds, and a medical committee, responsible for clinical activities, admissions policies, methods, and other medical aspects of the work. This was an example of "do what I say, not what I do," as Sanger, a lay woman, was still in charge of all aspects of the BCCRB's work.[37]

Though many of the BCCRB's standards were similar to those of the ABCL, Sanger's group de-emphasized the organizational aspects of ABCL's affiliation. They did not ask for dues. They also put less emphasis on doctors' roles, though they argued that the physician was the ultimate authority in patient care. BCCRB affiliates were advised to have a medical advisory board "whenever possible," but most matters of clinic organization, fees, services, and regulations were left to local reformers to decide.[38] As Sanger suggested to her subordinates, "Affiliation does not mean dictating to these clinics, but is designed to assist them and give them the value of the material and data that we have collected on fifty thousand patients."[39]

The ABCL clinical standards focused on the clinic's relationship to the medical profession. They required clinics to have medical boards and excluded for-profit clinics. To ensure that clinics did not interfere with private medical practitioners, they recommended refusing patients who could afford physicians. Eric Matsner characterized the BCCRB's sliding scale of fees based upon patient income as a "racket" because they took fees as high as fifteen dollars.[40] The ABCL hoped that their clinic standards would encourage doctors to participate in the movement. The ABCL advised that the era of "the one-man clinic" was ending, to be replaced by "community enterprises" where groups of doctors would determine "admission requirements, fees, materials and equipment, hours, days, choice of clinicians, the relation of clinic to private practice, observers' privileges, follow-up, [and] record keeping." They wanted these medical committees to replace lay women as the chief interpreters of the birth control movement. In their eagerness to associate with medical men, the lay women at the ABCL did not seem concerned that they were writing themselves out of their own movement.[41]

The competition between ABCL affiliation and BCCRB certification must have seemed like a tempest in a teapot to those not directly engaged in it. Both accused the other of poaching. Sanger attacked the ABCL on its ability to actually provide information for the clinics. "The way that any national organization can be useful to a state organization is by making it possible for lecturers, speakers, field workers and other assistants help to build up constructive state development," she wrote, then claiming "the American Birth Control League has practically no Research Committee nor facilities where the local clinics might be advised as they can be at our Clinical Research Bureau."[42] From the ABCL's perspective, Sanger was the interloper, creating duplication and confusion in the movement with her copycat program. In a bitter letter to British physician Maurice Newfield, Eric Matsner charged that once Sanger had secured the *One Package* decision and closed the NCFLBC, she turned to clinic expansion, which had always been of "secondary" concern to her. He argued that she used NCFLBC field workers to "affiliate as many of the already established centers throughout the country as possible."[43] In fact, both organizations had worked to establish clinics throughout the 1930s; what was different in 1935 was that both wanted to lead this field and neither would willingly cede their stake. If clinics could choose between affiliations, the ABCL feared that they might prefer Sanger's option, not just because of her name recognition, but because she required less and offered more. She, in turn, believed that local activists would do what worked best in their own cities and tried to offer them more in terms of cooperation than control.

National organizations like the ABCL and the BCCRB hoped to direct the development of birth control clinics. By targeting certain areas for field work, providing networking opportunities, and developing guidelines for clinical practice, the national movement hoped to influence local activists and train them to see the movement as they wanted. There were differences between the two organizations; each approached their leadership roles from different perspectives, but both aimed to make the clinic experience similar no matter where a patient lived. Standards and guidelines developed for the clinic administrator, the organizing group, the staff and physicians at the clinic, along with a white list of contraceptive methods; these were the first steps in trying to achieve these commonalities. But did they work?

The View from the Clinic

Operating a birth control clinic was necessarily local work. Clinic activists' first goal was to serve the women in their city, sometimes even in just one neighborhood. The national movement played an important role in their work, but I would argue that its chief role was that of inspiration. Without the national birth control movement, or the work of Margaret Sanger, there would not have been local leagues and there would not have been clinics. But once the inspiration had taken root, the clinic activists did not need the national movement nearly as much as the national movement needed them.

Once a clinic was operational, all the impediments to its success were local. They needed to attract sufficient financial support, secure facilities that were reliable and inexpensive, and win the support of key medical, political, and social figures in their vicinity. They needed to be able to attract and keep their patients, and they needed volunteers or paid staff to treat them. National activists and organizations could not help with these issues. They operated on a larger stage, one of changing public perceptions about birth control, rewriting outdated morality laws, and encouraging the medical profession and the government to accept responsibility for the health of the nation's women and children. All the arguments, articles, speeches, and testimonies produced by the national organizations raised the local activists' consciousness about issues of race, ethnicity, women's emancipation and health, the eugenic value of the population, and the economic system that produced the poverty they hoped to alleviate. But even if the local activists accepted these arguments, to be of any use such concepts had to be tested in the crucible of the clinic. Was a particular practice or approach beneficial to the patients they treated? Did it help attract more patients? Did it alienate potential supporters? Would it bring the ire of the local medical society or church groups? Did it make sense given local social relations?

The clinics got more than they gave to the national movement. They were provided expert advice and assistance, occasional financial support, and access to less-expensive supplies. They were sometimes able to lure nationally prominent figures like Margaret Sanger to attract attention to their activities, and they were given a community of other leagues and clinics and a rationale to rally around. But little was asked back, and even that little was often begrudged. Clinics were resolutely independent from the national organizations and leaders, rejecting efforts to control or tithe them, and backing away from any binding relationships.

The national organizations (even in the 1920s, when the ABCL was the only one), had no power over local leagues and clinics. They could refuse to include them on their national registers of clinics. They could refuse to certify or affiliate them, but as censure goes, they were not much of a threat. This was before the day when "Planned Parenthood" had become a brand. Clinics in the 1920s and 1930s called themselves "Birth Control Clinics," "Maternal Health Clinics," "Family Relations Centers," "Sex Hygiene Services," or "Mothers' Clinics." Whether or not a clinic cooperated with the national organizations had little effect on its popularity with patients or local social leaders. Local concerns always trumped national ones.

An instance in Indianapolis provides a good example of the independence of local organizers. Clarence Gamble, an ABCL and BCCRB board member, sent field organizer Elsie Wulkop to Indianapolis to help establish a birth control clinic in 1932. The Indianapolis Maternal Health Clinic's new medical committee ignored Wulkop's advice and drafted a draconian admissions policy: to be seen, a woman had to have been married at least two years, have at least two children, be referred from a social worker or physician, *and* be unable to pay a private physician. The medical committee felt that such rules were needed to placate the Indianapolis Medical Society. When Wulkop protested, they suggested that they might "change these rules very shortly after the clinic is opened." Gamble's entreaties could not convince them to liberalize the admissions policy either. They rejected his request to accept any married woman without regard to how many children she had. In this case, Gamble did have some power over the fledgling clinic, as he threatened to withdraw the funding he had offered the clinic. But the Maternal Health Clinic's Medical Committee remained committed to their decision. Faced with this implacable resistance, Gamble blinked, providing the funds. Shortly afterward another rift rose between them. Gamble wanted the clinic to advertise broadly to bring large numbers of patients, but the Maternal Health League preferred to maintain a low-key operation to avoid opposition. This also ended badly for Gamble. Reading through the Indianapolis league's board minutes, one finds frequent references to the national organization and to Gamble, but both seemed mostly to be distant pressures that could be easily ignored. What Clarence Gamble, Elsie Wulkop, or the ABCL thought of their clinic was not nearly as important as the perceptions of the Indianapolis Medical Society, local politicians, or women's groups. The Indianapolis league, like most leagues, refused to pay the dues that the ABCL recommended. Each time this appeal was brought up at board meetings, the board would dryly note that they were only "nominally affiliated" with the league and move on to the next issue.[44]

Many local activists were more politically and socially conservative than national leaders, especially Margaret Sanger. Many preferred to keep their relations with the national birth control leagues, especially in the 1920s, on an unofficial basis. In Chicago, the IBCL's relationship with the Chicago Woman's Aid Society was far more important and critical to its success than was its relations with the ABCL. The IBCL generally kept itself at arm's reach from the ABCL, highlighting its independence from the New York organization. In other cities, clinics that tried to secure funding from civic organizations like the Community Chest found that they were better served if they were seen as local maternal health services, not as affiliates of Sanger's BCCRB or the ABCL. And though it faded in importance throughout the 1930s, there was a real medical prejudice against associating with Margaret Sanger that led many clinics' medical advisors, as in Indianapolis, to set their clinic apart and demonstratively reject her policies as too lenient.[45]

The CMHA long refused to ally with any national association, claiming that it was not interested in legislative programs and it feared that the national movement's tactics and propaganda were likely to alienate potential donors and create "opposition from religious and racial groups." The Cleveland activists saw themselves as a local charity that was stronger without any national entanglements, a stand they maintained until 1942, when they finally affiliated with the PPFA.[46] Most hospital clinics felt the same. Few had any direct or regular contact with lay birth control leaders. Sanger herself agreed that the relationship between local organizations and the national movement was an odd fit. In 1939 she wrote BCFA executive director Kenneth Rose: "In my opinion, you cannot organize a national organization around local issues. Our national organization [the NCFLBC] had interests centered in Washington, getting a bill passed. It's quite a different matter to have a national organization set up for sponsoring local clinics."[47]

Most local clinics joined national organizations out of loyalty to those who had helped them organize. For many founded in the 1920s and early 1930s, Margaret Sanger held a special place in their clinic's history. The first generation of pioneers, who founded leagues and opened clinics, often demonstrated a personal loyalty to Sanger that clinic activists in the 1930s were less likely to express. When, after Sanger's resignation from the ABCL in 1928, the ABCL asked Hilda Cornish to affiliate her Little Rock Birth Control Clinic with it, she immediately consulted Sanger. Cornish feared that affiliating with the ABCL would jeopardize her relationship with Sanger. Sanger was critical of the ABCL's ability to offer Little Rock much, but did not tell Cornish to refuse them, and the Arkansas league did eventually affiliate. But by the mid-1930s the field workers who helped start clinics were not as famous as Sanger, and though the local leaders welcomed them, they felt no difficulty in overruling them.[48]

Neither the ABCL's affiliation program nor the BCCRB's certification offer were wildly successful, another demonstration of the limits of national control over local clinics. In the race to gather affiliates, the ABCL was more successful, though they admitted that the response was "immediate, but not overwhelming." Only about 35 percent of clinics joined in the first year (159 of a possible 450), despite the fact that this effort was the ABCL's chief goal that year. Over the next few years the figure rose slowly, but never reached 55 percent. The BCCRB had even less success, with only 98 clinics certified by the middle of 1936.[49] Their effort was poorly timed and organized, launched just before Sanger left on a three-month tour of India. Though Sanger thought the program "one of the most important and progressive steps in the birth control movement," she feared that it would fail if it were not staffed appropriately. BCCRB secretary Hazel Zborowski reported that Hannah Stone seemed content with merely sending the *JOC* to the affiliated clinics, while she thought that "much more is needed. These clinics should be personally contacted in some way so that their problems could be handled and their affiliation of some value beside just having the name of belonging to the Clinical Research Bureau group."[50] While the BCCRB undertook more widespread information dissemination through the clinic reports published in the *JOC* and through the Conference on Contraceptive Research and Clinical Practice organized in December 1936, the affiliation program as a whole did not prosper.[51]

From the point of view of the clinic, the affiliation war held little interest. Many independent clinics hedged their bets, affiliating with both organizations. Most institutional clinics didn't affiliate with either, though the ABCL format appealed to some hospital clinics. For many, affiliation simply formalized benefits that they already received from the ABCL and BCCRB. It is unlikely that either program conferred the stature the league hoped it would, and there is no indication that patients, doctors, or the local community were aware of the honor, or used it to determine whether they could trust a clinic.

Clinic activists always looked more to building and maintaining the fragile coalitions between local groups than they did working on a solid relationship with the national movement. Many of their decisions worked against the national goals, such as their penchant for keeping their work under the radar. Most eschewed newspaper reports of their work, fearing that it might alert Catholics and other opponents to their existence. Over time this fear began to fade, as clinic after clinic found that the occasional public interest story not only increased donations, but brought them new patients as well. Even when clinics did draw the ire of local clergymen or moralists, few sought help from national organizations for fear that they might inflame the situation rather than soothe it. There were instances where a birth control exhibit was banned in a public fair and national leaders like Sanger would excoriate the government officials and religious leaders behind the ban, sometimes in ways that may have burned bridges for more cautious clinic activists. Once the hoopla was over, the national leaders left, and clinic activists were left to try to repair the damaged relationships with the powers that be. Sanger was well known for counseling heated and spirited resistance to any effort to censure or close clinics, encouraging language that, if used, could harden feelings. When they chose to respond in a more conciliatory manner, Sanger often disparaged clinic activists as timid and spineless. But the local activists usually had a better sense of the temperature of the city and knew what could be accomplished and what could not.[52]

Despite the efforts of national leaders and organizations to control the clinic movement, power at the birth control clinic remained in local hands. The head of a local league or clinic, such as the Indianapolis Maternal Health League, was an autonomous activist. She did not have to listen to the head of the state birth control league, nor follow the orders of the ABCL president or Margaret Sanger. The national movement attempted, over the course of the 1920s and 1930s, to create such hierarchies, but its efforts failed. At their core, birth control clinics were local organizations and control over them stayed on Main Street, where the funding, volunteers, and patients were to be found.

Conclusion

In 1930, the ABCL moved its offices to Madison Avenue, home to advertising agencies that shaped public perception and polished corporate images. It was an apt location, for by the end of the decade the national birth control movement was no longer in the business of providing birth control information to needy women. Instead, it advised and loosely directed the efforts of state affiliates, produced high-quality educational materials, and lobbied federal and state governments and medical associations for support. It held splashy annual meetings that made the news, reported on the increasing numbers of clinics and leagues, and patted itself contentedly on the back. On Madison Avenue, activists no longer intimately knew the women they strove to help; most had never seen their patients except in the photographs they selected to illustrate pamphlets about the benefits of a planned family. This was a far cry from the league's early days, when Sanger described her *Birth Control Review* office in 1918: "That little room is a blessing to womankind. We have all our Board meetings there and during the past six months it has averaged twenty-five women a week coming there for advice. Some days ten or fifteen come. It's really a clinic only there is no noise about it."[1]

On Main Street, in cities all over the nation, the birth control activists who opened and operated over five hundred clinics were still working on the front lines. Their clinics had treated hundreds of thousands of women. Activists, patients, and clinicians all shared the clinic's physical space. By their sheer numbers, these local activists, working in leagues and clinics, vastly outnumbered the score of activists who worked in the New York headquarters. Most clinics relied on twenty to fifty activists for support; they included doctors, nurses, clerical workers, medical and legal advisors, officers, directors, trustees, and donors. Multiplied by the number of clinics in operation, they numbered at least twenty-five thousand strong.

The work that these two groups of activists did was different. Clinic work remained rooted in the most fundamental aspects of the birth control cause. They provided contraceptive information and aid directly to the women who needed it. Yes, they also crafted brochures, ran annual fund-raising events, even lobbied local governments and medical groups to support their work, but day-in and day-out they interacted with the clinic. They saw firsthand both the need for and the benefit of their efforts. Whether manning the front desk, ordering or selling diaphragms and other supplies, or taking information from a nervous first-time patient, clinic activists had a far more personal connection to the birth control cause. It was this connection to the patients, their lives, and their care that kept the clinic activists fired up to support and expand the movement. In the offices on Madison Avenue, the link between activists and patients was stretched to the breaking point, if not long broken.

A successful movement for reproductive rights needed both national and local activists, but they did not function simply as leaders and followers. The national activists worked on the level of ideas; they developed and propagated arguments for birth control that appealed to broad segments of the population; they forged connections with other social and medical agencies to help the movement; and they inspired the creation of local leagues and clinics. Clinic activists operated at a different level. They picked and chose from the vast smorgasbord of ideas, rationales, and advice offered up by the national movement, always asking how they could use these ideas. Were they practical? Did they address the clinic's needs? If the answer was no, clinic activists ignored the suggestions, doing what had to be done to have a successful clinic in their town. Though the activists on Madison Avenue wanted to direct the development of the movement, their efforts failed, as activists on Main Street refused to slavishly follow their lead.

The emphasis shifts, in almost every way, if we shift the focus and look at the clinic as the center of birth control activism. Issues that were complex at the national level, like the relationship between birth control and eugenics, seem simpler at the clinic. While eugenic arguments for birth control might have appealed to activists, they could not work them in any practical way into the rules and routines of the clinic. Likewise, activists found it difficult to overcome racial prejudice when designing their clinics, focused as they were on creating a community organization. Very few clinics were integrated, a few more offered segregated services for African Americans, but the vast majority limited their services to whites.

Clinic activists preferred practical solutions to sweeping ideals or fighting stances. They did not want to establish themselves as confrontational or divisive. If at all possible, they would figure out how to work with and win over potential enemies, such as government officials, medical societies, churches, and newspapermen. If that meant that they treated fewer patients but faced less opposition, they found it a fair trade. Clinic activists had to live in the communities they served and so they avoided burning bridges behind them, preferring quiet persuasion instead of loud confrontation.

When Margaret Sanger founded the first birth control clinic in Brownsville, Brooklyn, in 1916, the clinic she created did not serve as the blueprint for the six hundred and fifty that followed. Activists were not certain whether it was best to pursue independent models, where they could control all aspects of the work, or institutional clinics within existing health and social organizations, which were better integrated into the local community. While the independent clinic was publicized most widely and successfully, it was never the only way to organize a clinic. From the very start, it competed with hospital-based clinics (in New York), settlement clinics (in Chicago), and early public health services (in California). None of these models were perfect, and each clinic group had to decide what it valued and what it could accomplish. If patient happiness was an activist's highest priority, she might prefer to create an independent or settlement clinic. If acceptance by the medical profession was paramount, the activist would work with the local hospital to offer the services. And if the reduction of maternal and infant death rates were the impetus for the clinic, the activist would be inclined to work in tandem with public health clinics. Even within these broad groupings, there were variations, as each activist put a unique stamp on what the clinic would do, who it would serve, and where it would be located.

If this book does nothing other than complicate the idea of what a birth control clinic was in the 1920s and 1930s, it will have enabled a better understanding of the roots of the reproductive rights movement. Birth control clinics were narrowly focused in the early years, both in regard to methods and patients. Over the course of the two decades, their services broadened to include marriage counseling, infertility treatments, and contraceptive research. They gradually opened their doors to more and different women. While early clinics targeted poor, married, urban immigrants, in the next twenty years clinics treated larger numbers of the American born, African

Americans, younger, and sometimes unmarried women. Though the older guard would resist, by the 1950s Planned Parenthood was advising the unmarried and teenagers in the hopes of thwarting an illegitimacy boom. And while the diaphragm was an overwhelming favorite among contraceptives at clinics, over time they experimented with other methods and eventually switched their allegiance to the birth control pill.

Looking inside the clinics, I have tried to provide a sense of how they operated, who worked in them, and why they were successful. The clinics that were popular combined a sympathetic space with a service that many women valued. They offered the very best contraceptive known, and while this method was not the most appealing, it was the contraceptive that the activists themselves would use. Though the clinic's advice might start with contraceptives, it seems clear that it did not stop there. Activists advised women on child rearing, marital relations, and access to other medical and social services. They did not satisfy every woman who came through their doors, but when the patient's desire to control her family was strong enough, and she was determined, the clinic's advice and methods were remarkably successful.

One important finding was that the gender patterns of activist participation documented at the national level did not hold true at the local level. National birth control organizations thought that male participation and leadership would improve the public perception of birth control and help secure the medical and governmental support that they sought for clinics. To meet their goals of fostering government-funded or medically based institutional clinics, they needed access to traditional avenues of power. They did not feel that lay women had that kind of access, and in the 1920s and early 1930s this lack of support seemed to harm efforts to broaden the movement. The male heads of hospitals and public health departments had proved unwilling to prioritize birth control, even as they criticized the independent clinics created by women. The national answer to the problem was to include more men in leadership positions in the belief that this was the key to being taken more seriously. Doctors like Eric Matsner and Richard Pierson directed the ABCL's tactics in the late 1930s, and as the organization entered the 1940s it began ushering in a series of short-term, medical or public health oriented, male presidents, officers, and directors.

At the local level, when activists were faced with the reality that neither hospitals nor public health departments would take on responsibility for birth control, lay women created independent clinics to meet the need. Though they wanted birth control to be integrated seamlessly into America's health care system, their chief commitment was to provide the service to their local community. Clinic activists would rather institute a less-perfect clinic today than lobby for years for the perfect one to be provided by the government or a hospital. Lay women, so critical to the creation of the clinics, did not step back into the shadows. They continued to direct and operate the clinics, using men as advisors and clinicians when needed. For clinics, birth control organizing remained a task best done by women.

The twentieth century was the first century that offered most women the practical ability to control their fertility. The birth control movement—both in its national and local forms—created this ability. National activists built more respectable rationales for contraception—ones that rejected associations of immorality and free love in favor of improved maternal and infant health and economic advantage. Local clinics provided a nearby means for women to achieve that control. They served as a proving ground for contraceptives, for ideas about sex and marriage, and for questions of who could use contraceptives. For the three hundred thousand women who walked through clinic doors, they provided a service that could be life changing.

Clinics did not reach everyone who needed them. Because of their locations and rationales, they best served working-class women in urban areas. But there were many more potential patients. Rural women out of reach of medical services, middle-class women who were too shy to discuss the topic with their family physicians, women of color who felt unwelcome in a movement that seemed designed by and for white women—all of these women may never have used a clinic, but they knew that they existed. As birth control clinics popped up on the Main Streets of cities and towns across America, activists publicized their work and popularized the notion that there were times when a woman—any woman—might want to restrict her fertility. What was good for an indigent mother of seven could also, at times, be good for the new bride of a recent college graduate just getting started in a profession. Control over fertility was something that any woman could use; it was an essential first step to gaining control of other aspects of her life. The birth control clinics, begun in the 1920s, were the hub at which this information was transferred, a place where one could learn, as Margaret Sanger called, "what every mother should know."[2]

Notes

INTRODUCTION

1. Crystal Eastman, "Birth Control in the Feminist Program," *BCR* 2:1 (Jan. 1918): 3.

2. George Gallup, "The Gallup Poll: Birth Control Information through Public Health Clinics Favored in Survey," *Washington Post*, Jan. 24, 1940.

3. Ruth Crocker, *Social Work and Social Order: The Settlement Movement in Two Industrial Cities, 1889–1930* (Urbana: University of Illinois Press, 1992), 6.

4. Stix and Notestein, *Controlled Fertility*, and Kopp, *Birth Control in Practice*, both described the BCCRB. Ruth Robishaw's "Study of 4,000 Patients" documented the CMHA, while Regine K. Stix's three-part article, "Birth Control in a Midwestern City: A Study of the Clinics of the Cincinnati Committee of Maternal Health," described the Cincinnati Maternal Health Clinic (*Milbank Memorial Fund Quarterly* 7:1 [Jan. 1939]: 57–68; 7:2 [Apr. 1939]: 152–71; 7:4 [Oct. 1939]: 392–493). Robinson's *Seventy Birth Control Clinics* was the first interpretive summary of clinic work covering both the United States and Europe.

5. For examples, see Lewis and Young, "Baltimore's Negro Health Center," 94; Marsh, "Birth Control Centers in Settlements," 141–42; see also the series of "Clinic Reports" published in the *JOC*, including "Minnesota Birth Control League," 2:1 (Jan. 1937): 19–20, the "Greenwich Committee for Maternal Health," 2:6 (June 1937): 140, and "Birth Control Clinic Here Aims at Preservation of Maternal Health" (Wilmington, Del.) *Sunday Morning Star*, Apr. 18, 1937.

6. Chief among these are the Margaret Sanger Papers, available on microfilm (MSP-L, MSP-S, and MSP-C), the Clarence Gamble Papers (Gamble), and the Records of the Planned Parenthood Federation of America (PPFAR).

7. Gordon, *Moral Property*, 250–59; Meyer, "Birth Control Policy," 52–53.

8. Reed, *From Private Vice to Public Virtue*, 106–28; McCann, *Birth Control Politics*, 6.

9. Maria H. Anderson's history of the Maternal Health Center of Houston is "Private Voices vs. Public Choices: The History of Planned Parenthood in Houston"; Marianne Leung wrote "'Better Babies': The Arkansas Birth Control Movement during the 1930s"; Jimmy E. W. Meyer's work on the CMHA is *Any Friend of the Movement;* and Johanna Schoen's study of North Carolina is *Choice and Coercion.* Article-length profiles of local clinics and leagues include: Lindemeyer, "Expanding Birth Control"; Christine F. Nicoll and Robert Weisbord, "The Early Years of the Rhode Island Birth Control League," *Rhode Island History* 45 (Nov. 1986): 111–25; William B. Turner, "Class, Controversy, and Contraceptives: Birth Control Advocacy in Nashville, 1932–1944," *Tennessee Historical Quarterly* 53:3 (Fall 1994): 166–79; Haslett, "Hull House"; and Mary Losure, "'Motherhood Protection' and the Minnesota Birth Control League," *Minnesota History* 54:8 (Winter 1995): 359–70.

10. Caron, *Who Chooses?* 12–13.

11. Holz, "Birth Control Clinic," 77–79.

12. For those seeking a more detailed analysis, see Gordon, *Moral Property*, Reed, *From Private Vice to Public Virtue*, McCann, *Birth Control Politics*, and Caron, *Who Chooses?*

13. See J. A. Banks, *Prosperity and Parenthood: A Study of Family Planning among the Victorian Middle Class* (London: Routledge and Kegan Paul, 1954), and with Olive Banks, *Feminism and Family Planning in Victorian England* (Liverpool: Liverpool University Press, 1964) for early work explaining the demographic transition. See also Richard A. Soloway, *Birth Control and the Population Question in England, 1877–1930* (Chapel Hill: University of North Carolina Press, 1977); Brodie, *Contraception and Abortion;* and Robert Jütte, *Contraception: A History* (Malden, Mass.: Polity, 2008), 106–56.

14. For further details, see Brodie, *Contraception and Abortion*, Tone, *Devices and Desires*, and James F. Cooper, *Technique of Contraception* (New York: Day-Nichols, 1928).

15. The contraceptive market grew rapidly, fueled by changes in the structure and meaning of the family and the beginnings of a mass consumer culture that brought products otherwise unavailable to small towns and villages via mail-order catalogs (see Brodie, *Contraception and Abortion*, 232–42, and Tone, *Devices and Desires*, 85–87).

16. In the United States, many of the authors of such works also provided information in public lectures that included general discussions of male and female anatomy and hygiene. Some of these lectures were given by women, and occasionally the speaker had some medical training. For more on this phenomenon, see Brodie, *Contraception and Abortion*, chap. 4.

17. Brodie, *Contraception and Abortion*, 180–82 and 281–86.

18. Comstock's impact is detailed in Beisel, *Imperiled Innocents*, 199–201.

19. Brodie, *Contraception and Abortion*, 281–86.

20. Aletta Jacobs, *Memories: My Life as an International Leader in Health, Suffrage, and Peace* (New York: Feminist Press, trans. 1996), 49.

21. Rosanna Ledbetter, *History of the Malthusian League, 1877–1927* (Columbus: University of Ohio Press, 1976), 178–80.

22. For Sanger's early career and relations with Goldman, see Katz, *Selected Papers* 1:69–71 and 93–97.

23. Alice Wexler, *Emma Goldman: An Intimate Life* (New York: Pantheon Books, 1984), 209–16; Sanger, *Autobiography*, 203–7.

24. Pessaries were marketed as "womb supporters" to get around legal restrictions on contraceptives. See Sanger, *My Fight*, 150–58.

25. Martin, "'Police Can't Stop Me.'"

26. Sanger and Byrne's trials garnered headlines in New York and other cities, especially when Ethel Byrne went on a hunger strike while imprisoned at Blackwell's Island (Martin,"'Police Can't Stop Me'"; for more details see Sanger, *Autobiography*, 213–19, and Katz, *Selected Papers* 1:194–220).

27. Originally called the Clinical Research Department, after its split with the ABCL

Sanger renamed it the Birth Control Clinical Research Bureau. In 1940 it became the Margaret Sanger Research Bureau, and in 1973 took the name Planned Parenthood of New York City. For simplicity's sake, I have used the BCCRB throughout this book to refer to Sanger's clinic.

28. Sanger, *My Fight*, 281–99.

29. See Katz, *Selected Papers* 1:420–22.

30. John Price Jones Corporation, "Survey and Plan of Fund-Raising for the BCCRB and the NCFLBC," Sept. 15, 1930 (MSP-S 61:476); ABCL Board of Directors Minutes, Nov. 3, 1932 (PPLMR) and May 23, 1935 (MSP-L 33).

31. The percentage ranged between 5 and 25 percent of a local league's contributions. ABCL, Board of Directors Minutes, Sept. 11, 1928, Oct. 5, 1933, and Jan. 20, 1932 (MSP-S 61:135, MSP-L 28:07, and PPLMR).

32. See Pringle, "What Do the Women of America Think?" 14.

33. See Katz, *Selected Papers* 2:203–5 and 303.

34. ABCL Board of Directors, Feb. 8, 1934, Mar. 17, 1934, and Apr. 38, 1935 (MSP-L 28:24–30).

35. NCFLBC, *New Day Dawns*, 37; NCFLBC, "Rough Notes on Meeting," Apr. 23, 1937 (MSP-S 64:601).

36. McCann, *Birth Control Politics*, 191.

37. Eric Matsner, Annual Report of the ABCL Medical Department for 1937 (PPFAR); Minutes of Birth Control Council of America, June 22, 1937 (MSP-S 62:16).

38. A Joint Committee of the ABCL and BCCRB met in July 1938 to try again. After determining that the two organizations were "so similar that duplication of effort developed almost all along the line," merger plans began, concluding in January 1939 (ABCL Annual Report, 1938 [PPFAR]).

39. Sanger to Robert Latou Dickinson, Jan. 24, 1939 (MSP-C 6:962).

40. Widowed in 1943, Sanger returned to prominence after World War II, but starred largely on the international stage, as the founding president of the International Planned Parenthood Federation (Chesler, *Woman of Valor*, 399–413).

41. See Chesler, *Woman of Valor*, 435–40.

CHAPTER 1: BIRTH CONTROL CLINIC MODELS

1. The aggregate data used here was gathered from documents such as national clinic directories, lists, and reports created by birth control leagues, as well as pamphlets, letters, and other ephemera of the birth control movement. For information on the methods used to record and analyze these documents see http://www.press.uillinois.edu/books/hajo/appendix.php.

2. ABCL Annual Report, 1937 (PPFAR).

3. The government clinics include 62 clinics founded between 1937 and 1939 in North Carolina rural public health departments. While these clinics made up almost 12 percent of the 404 clinics operating in the United States, over a two-year period only 1,311 patients were treated in all 62 clinics (an average of 10.5 patients per year per clinic). By contrast, the BCCRB treated approximately fifteen thousand patients a year ("Prevenceptive Centers in Whole-Time City, County, and District

Health Departments, North Carolina State Board of Health," Mar. 15, 1937-Mar. 15, 1939 [Weil]; Sanger to Norman E. Himes, June 25, 1931; see also BCCRB General Summary, Year Ending Nov. 30, 1935 [MSP-C 5:217 and S 61:807]).

4. Sanger to BCCRB worker M. Frances Warren, Jan. 13, 1932 (MSP-L 32:456).

5. Martin, "'Police Can't Stop Me'" (quotes 1 and 2). Thygeson could not recall exactly when the St. Paul clinic was founded, but it was after Sanger's 1916 visit to the city (Sherna Gluck, ed., *From Parlor to Prison: Five American Suffragists Talk about their Lives* [New York: Octagon Books, 1976], 50–53, quotes 3 and 4).

6. Sanger, *My Fight*, 191.

7. Indianapolis Maternal Health League, Board of Directors Minutes, 1932–34, and the 1938 Annual Report (PPCIR).

8. "Eugenic" reasons referred to fears of hereditary physical or mental defects. "Social reasons" usually referred to abusive, criminal, or alcoholic spouses. Medical indications included conditions that were exacerbated during pregnancy, such as tuberculosis, kidney disease, or heart problems (see the Indiana Maternal Health League Annual Report, 1938 [PPCIR]; Elsa Haerle, "Annual Report of the Maternal Health League of Indiana, to the ABCL," 1936 [PPFAR]).

9. Elizabeth Walsh, "Spreading the News," *BCR* 9:6 (June 1926): 192; Battle Creek Maternal Health Association, 1934–35 Report, and Monroe County Birth Control League, "Report of the Rochester County Maternal Consultation Centers," Feb. 1937 (PPASLR); Meyer, "Birth Control Policy," 215.

10. Anderson, "Private Choices," 69; Marguerite Martin, "In Behalf of Mothers," *St. Louis Post-Dispatch*, Mar. 31, 1937.

11. A smaller number of clinics were located in churches, but there is insufficient documentation to draw any conclusions.

12. Pennsylvania Birth Control Federation Flyer, ca. 1934 (MSP-L 103:759).

13. Birth Control League of Delaware, Annual Report to the ABCL, 1936 (PPFAR); San Joaquin General Hospital Clinic to Cele Damon, Dec. 23, 1936, and George Cooper to Leo Heller, Oct. 30, 1939 (MSP-L 33:704 and 18:167); Guttmacher, *Planned Parenthood Beginnings*, 109.

14. "Waterbury Clinic Report," June 27, 1939 (PPFAR).

15. Sanger's reaction to the "rumpus" in North Carolina was bemusement, writing to her secretary, "It will soon be the period of the Stone Age in other words—when the leaders and the pioneers will begin to be stoned" (George M. Cooper to Sanger, Feb. 8, 1938, and Sanger to Florence Rose, Feb. 1, 1938 [MSP-S 14:382 and 344]).

16. Lindemeyer, "Expanding Birth Control," 169–71.

17. Don Wharton, "Birth Control: The Case for the State," *Atlantic Monthly*, Oct. 1939, 465.

18. Stevens, *In Sickness and In Wealth*, 105–39.

19. Meckel, *Save the Babies*, 217. For more on the medical profession and preventive medicine, see Ellen S. More, *Restoring the Balance: Women Physicians and the Professionalization of Medicine, 1850–1995* (Cambridge: Harvard University Press, 2001), 161, and Robin L. Rosen, "Federal Expansion, Fertility Control, and Physicians in

the United States: The Politics of Motherhood in the Interwar Years," *Journal of Women's History* 10:3 (Aug. 1998): 60–61.

20. Stevens, *In Sickness and In Wealth*, 136; the quoted text is a description of the Cook County Hospital in Chicago.

21. Stevens, *In Sickness and In Wealth*, 49; Robinson, *Seventy Birth Control Clinics*, 26 (quote); James F. Cooper, *Technique of Contraception* (New York: Day Nichols, 1928), 217–19; Robert Dickinson to Anne Kennedy, ca. 1925 (MSP-L 32:104).

22. The clinics at Mount Sinai Hospital and the Lenox Hill Hospital accepted patients from "any legal source," but they got few referrals from in-house physicians, many of whom were unaware that the hospital provided the service (McCann, *Birth Control Politics*, 80; Robinson, *Seventy Birth Control Clinics*, 123–24 [quote]).

23. Ruth Topping, Memo to Bureau of Social Hygiene Files, Mar. 27, 1931 (BSHR).

24. Robinson, *Seventy Birth Control Clinics*, 26; McCann, *Birth Control Politics*, 80–81; Louise Stevens Bryant, "Report of the Executive Secretary," Mar. 9, 1926 (NCMHR); Robert Dickinson to Clarence Little, Oct. 22, 1925 (MSP-L 32:17 [quote]); and Sanger, *My Fight*, 315.

25. The admission policy in Cincinnati was broader than that in New York, and the fact that it was the only birth control clinic in Cincinnati also contributed to its success. In 1930, two more clinics were founded, at the Jewish Hospital, and at a settlement house (Robert Latou Dickinson, "Medical Aspects of Human Fertility," 1930 [NCMHR], 26; Lindemeyer, "Expanding Birth Control," 165–71; Guttmacher, *Planned Parenthood Beginnings*, 101).

26. Stevens, *In Sickness and In Wealth*, 140–44. Another clinic that followed this model was the Pasadena Woman's Hospital Clinic.

27. Garrow, *Liberty and Sexuality*, 8.

28. Detroit Woman's Hospital Maternal Health Clinic, "Resume of Cases from Apr. 8th, 1931 to Aug. 31st, 1932" (PPLDR); Lamport, "Recreation Rooms," 36–39; Dickinson and Morris, "Birth Control Centers."

29. Robinson, *Seventy Birth Control Clinics*, 123–24, 129.

30. Rev. Rufus D. S. Putney to Clara Louise McGraw, Mar. 21, 1932 (PPASLR).

31. Rodrique, "Afro-American Community," 211 n. 45.

32. San Joaquin General Hospital Clinic to Cele Damon, Dec. 23, 1936 (MSP-L 33:704).

33. See Gamble for voluminous correspondence between Gamble, Donald West (his representative), and Hospital Board chair Florence Banning, especially Gamble to West, Nov. 29, 1933, and Jan. 9, 1934; West to Gamble, Aug. 2 and 10, 1933, Sept. 5, 1933, Oct. 24, 1933, and Nov. 19, 1933; and Banning to West, Nov. 7 and 17, 1933 (Gamble).

34. Marsh, "Birth Control Centers," 141.

35. Chicago Women's Aid Society, Reports of the Birth Control Committee, Apr. 16, 1929, and Apr. 18, 1933 (CWASR); Haslett, "Hull House," 263–69; Guttmacher, *Planned Parenthood Beginnings*, 40–41.

36. Chicago Woman's Aid Society, Reports of the Birth Control Committee,

1928–39; Muriel Harris to Mrs. Samuel Hirsch, Oct. 17, 1939, and Mar. 21, 1940 (CWASR).

37. Nash, "Planned Parenthood."

38. Forty percent of all settlements were found in three cities: New York, Boston, and Chicago (Allen F. Davis, "Settlement Houses," in Eric Foner and John A. Garraty, eds., *Reader's Companion to American History* [New York: Houghton Mifflin, 1991], 983–84).

39. Trolander, *Professionalism and Social Change*, 2; Allen F. Davis, *Spearheads for Reform: The Social Settlements and the Progressive Movement, 1840–1914* (New Brunswick, N.J.: Rutgers University Press, 1984), 230.

40. Trolander, *Professionalism and Social Change*, 23–34. Marsh, "Birth Control Centers" 141–42.

41. Natalie Lamport, "Report of Birth Control Work of the Recreation Rooms and Settlement Branch Birth Control Clinic Maternal Health Center," Mar. 1935 (MSP-L 32:312).

42. The Health Department had many other responsibilities as well, including the control of contagious disease, sanitary inspection of homes and food processing plants, and the provision of clean milk. For more on Pomeroy, see *NatCAB*, vol. 30 (New York: J. T. White and Co., 1943), 61; *Los Angeles Times*, Mar. 25, 1941; and Worchester, "Public Health and Private Doctors," 151.

43. Mexican infant mortality rates fell to 185/1000, still high, but a decline of 37 percent from 1915. Infant mortality figures among whites and Japanese and other ethnic groups were as low as 23/100, which compared with the best obtained worldwide (John L. Pomeroy, "Health Centers Valuable," *Los Angeles Times*, Oct. 21, 1928).

44. Robinson, *Seventy Birth Control Clinics*, 33–34; Kavinoky, "California Public Health and Mothers' Clinics," 205–7; Kavinoky to Sanger, June 18, 1934 (MSP-L 85:635), and Oct. 21, 1937 (MSP-S 13:635).

45. See Kavinoky's comment in Sanger and Stone, *Practice of Contraception*, 30.

46. For the Health Center procedures, see Pomeroy, "Los Angeles County Health Department Bureau of Medical and Social Service—Division of Clinics and Emergency Hospitals Mothers' Clinic," Feb. 21, 1930 (PPFAR), and Kavinoky, "California Public Health and Mothers' Clinics."

47. Kavinoky to Sanger, Dec. 6, 1933 (MSP-L 85:632).

48. The substance of the debate is published in Pomeroy, *Public Health;* see also Worchester, "Public Health and Private Doctors."

49. See Los Angeles County Medical Association Report, n.d., in Pomeroy, *Public Health*, 179; Harry Wiley et al., "Medical Bureau's Report on Health Centers," and John L. Pomeroy, "Report of the Huntington Park Public Health Program," July 31, 1931, in Pomeroy, *Public Health*, 72 and 62. For the mothers' clinics, see Kavinoky to Sanger, Oct. [?] 1931 (MSP-L 57:95), Dec. 6, 1933 (MSP-L 85:632), and Oct. 21, 1937 (MSP-S 13:635); Kavinoky to Clarence J. Gamble, Feb. 24, 1934 (Gamble). For the Health Department in general, see *Los Angeles Times*, June 23, 1931; Mar. 16, July 14, and July 28, 1932; Feb. 28, May 30, and Nov. 29, 1933; and Feb. 17, 1934.

50. Worchester, "Public Health and Private Doctors," 202–3.

51. ABCL Annual Report, 1937 (PPFAR). I have only been able to identify forty-eight government-sponsored clinics in 1937, likely a discrepancy between the number of clinics reported opened in North Carolina and the aggregate numbers claimed by the state. They reported that ninety-three counties were offering contraceptive services at their health centers, but did not give any names or locations. I located only fifty-two specific centers. The five states that were offering contraceptives were likely North Carolina, South Carolina, Florida, Virginia, and West Virginia (BCFA Program for 1942, Jan. 28, 1942 [MSP-L 113:494]; Schoen, *Choice and Coercion*, 60).

52. ABCL Annual Reports, 1936 and 1937 (PPFAR); Pope, "Story of Birth Control in Michigan."

53. Michigan Maternal Health League, Annual Report to the American Birth Control League, 1936 (PPFAR).

54. The longevity of these clinics is based upon their inclusion in national lists, which are more likely to report clinics as active after they had closed than to remove them if they were still operating. There are few documents in the records of the birth control movement that provide finite information about clinic closures, or reveal the reasons why most closed.

55. See Schoen, *Choice and Coercion*, chapter 1, for detailed coverage of this program.

56. Cooper, "Four Years of Contraception."

57. George M. Cooper to Leo Heller, Oct. 30, 1939 (MSP-L 118:167); North Carolina State Board of Health, "Prevenceptive Centers"; Cooper et al., "Four Years of Contraception"; Schoen, *Choice and Coercion*, 40–44; Gordon, *Moral Property*, 233.

58. Of the 1,311 patients attending the North Carolina clinics, a large percentage received advice only one time (565 patients, or 43 percent), while 46 patients reported failures (3.5 percent, slightly higher than most traditional birth control clinics found). Thirty eight patients complained of irritation (North Carolina State Board of Health, "Prevenceptive Centers in Whole-Time City, County and District Health Departments," Mar. 15, 1937–Mar. 15, 1939 [Norton]).

59. Gamble's initial investment was to have covered only one year, but he was persuaded to extend it until 1940. While patient counts climbed slowly in the 1940s, they declined dramatically by the late 1950s (Schoen, *Choice and Coercion*, 263 n. 139; Williams and Williams, *Every Child a Wanted Child*, 128–48; see also J. W. Roy Norton, "Twenty-One Years Experience with a Public Health Contraceptive Service," *American Journal of Public Health* 49:8 [Aug. 1959]: 993–1000).

60. While Sanger was not directly involved in the Gamble-funded public health clinics, her field workers had been in North Carolina since 1932 and the ABCL had sent organizers from 1935 to 1937 (Roy Norton, "A Health Department Birth Control Program," *American Public Health Association Journal* 29:3 [Mar. 1939]: 253–56; "North Carolina Leads the Way," *BCR* 22:12 [Dec. 1938]: 143–44; Hazel Moore to Florence Rose, Jan. 20, 1938 [MSP-L 118:163]; Ella Waddill to Roy Norton, Sept. 10, 1938 [Norton]; and "Under the Dome," *Raleigh News and Observer*, Jan. 15, 1938 [quote]).

61. Rodrique, "Afro-American Community," 199–200; Seibels, "Pregnancy Spacing" (quote).

CHAPTER 2: INSIDE THE BIRTH CONTROL CLINIC

1. Sanger, *Woman and the New Race*, 94.

2. For examples of the rationales developed for birth control, see Sanger, "When Should a Woman Avoid Having Children?" *BCR* 2:11 (Nov. 1918): 6–7; Sanger, "Case for Birth Control," Feb. 23, 1924; and "What Birth Control Can Do for India," Nov. 20, 1935 (MSP-S 70:759, MSP-C 16:212, 384).

3. Marjorie Prevost to Sanger, Feb. 26, 1932 (MSP-L 32:229).

4. Between 1934 and 1935, the BCCRB refused admission to 190 women. In some cases, such as when the woman was menstruating, the visit was merely postponed (Robinson, *Seventy Birth Control Clinics*, 70; BCCRB General Summary, Nov. 1934–Nov. 1935 [MSP-L 9:981]).

5. The Los Angeles Mothers' Clinic was also limited by law to offer contraception to "preserve life and prevent disease" (Tasker, "Mothers' Clinic," 252; Vreeland, "Process of Reform," Appendix on California Leagues, 365–68).

6. Dickinson and Morris, "Birth Control Centers," 591–93.

7. The ABCL reported that condoms were prescribed in 69 of 170 clinics, according to a 1937 survey, in a bit under 4 percent of cases. By 1939, the BCFA reported that only 1.6 percent of clinic patients were prescribed condoms (ABCL, Annual Report for 1937 [PPFAR]; Dickinson and Morris, "Birth Control Centers," 593).

8. For Sanger's views on male responsibility for birth control, see *Family Limitation*, 9–10, and *Woman and the New Race*, 96–98.

9. Mary Hughston, "Profiles of Tucson Mother's Clinic Patients," July 25, 1935 (MSP-L 83:564).

10. Leung, "'Better Babies,'" 80–81.

11. For example, Catholic activists used a range of attacks when testifying against the NCFLBC's proposed federal birth control bill. Ralph Burton attacked activists as "catspaws" of Russia, who sought to introduce free love and the abolishment of marriage through contraception. William Montavon claimed that birth control propaganda would pervert youth, while Dr. Henry W. Cattell argued that contraceptives would lure youth into premarital sex and later to abortion (U.S. Senate, *Birth Control Hearings before a Subcommittee of the Committee on the Judiciary, S. 4582, Feb. 13–14, 1931* [Washington, D.C.: GPO, 1931], 28, 30, and 60; for a detailed history of the Catholic opposition to birth control, see Leslie Tentler, *Catholics and Contraception: An American History* [Ithaca, N.Y.: Cornell University Press, 2004] and Tom Davis, *Sacred Work: Planned Parenthood and its Clergy Alliances* [New Brunswick, N.J.: Rutgers University Press, 2005]).

12. This happened in Salem, Massachusetts, where the decoy, an unmarried undercover police officer, may have feared that her fraud would be discovered during the gynecological examination. When married police officers attempted to infiltrate clinics under false names and identities, they were uniformly successful, and were

prescribed diaphragms (Lucille Lord-Heinstein, "The Salem Raid and Trial," *JOC* 2:6–7 [Aug.–Sept., 1937]: 156–57; Garrow, *Liberty and Sexuality*, 24–25.

13. The 1937 clinic figures are from "Summary of Reports from 170 Clinical Centers for 1937," ABCL Annual Report, 1937 (PPFAR). A sampling of individual clinics in the 1920s and early 1930s showed that patients averaged between four and six children, while by 1939 the BCFA reported an average of only 2.67 children (Los Angeles Mothers' Clinic, Survey of 3,000 Cases, Apr. 19, 1929, and Philadelphia Maternal Health Center, Annual Report, 1931 [MSP-L 85:656 and 31:332]; Meyer, *Any Friend*, 85; "Clinic Reports: Birth Control Educational Center," *JOC* 3:3 [Mar. 1938]: 68; Dickinson and Morris, "Birth Control Centers," 591–93).

14. Nash, "Planned Parenthood," 128–29.

15. Charles S. Higley, "Clinic Reports: Men's Consultation in a Maternal Health Center." *JOC* 2:10 (Oct. 1937): 187–88.

16. Stone, "Notes on a Roundtable Discussion"; Carol Nash, "Clinic Reports: Mothers' Health Center of the New York City Committee," *JOC* 2:4 (Apr. 1937): 91–92; National Clinic list, June 1935 (MSP-L 43:594).

17. Nash, "Planned Parenthood," 128–29.

18. Brownsville clinic flyer, ca. Oct. 1916 (MSP-S 62:835).

19. Women who were not pregnant often had irregular menses, sometimes caused by structural anomalies, but in many cases by the onset of menopause. In 1934 the BCCRB's "overdue clinic" saw four hundred potentially pregnant women. As word spread that there was no abortion assistance provided, the number of attendees declined dramatically (MS to Hannah Stone, Jan. 31, 1933, Lena Levine, "The Ascheim and Zondek Test," n.d., and Margaret Sanger, "Diagnostic Clinic policy," Jan. 28, 1934 [MSP-L 32:381, 752B, and 467]).

20. Los Angeles Mothers' Clinic, "Suggestions," n.d. (Noel); Haslett, "Hull House," 265; Sanger, "Why Not Birth Control Clinics in America?" *American Medicine* 3:5 (Mar. 1919): 164–67.

21. In a curt letter refusing to perform a therapeutic abortion, Dr. A. J. Walscheid of the Broad Street Hospital, "found no toxicosis or eclampsia, normal urine, no Bright's Disease or nephritis, no retinal damage from prior pregnancy, normal heart, lungs and blood pressure" (Walscheid to BCCRB, May 10, 1933 [MSP-L 32:408]).

22. Penelope B. P. Huse, "Confidential Report to Executive Committee," Dec. 1929 (PPFAR).

23. Dr. Siegal was likely Benjamin Segal, the husband of BCCRB clinician, Cheri Appel (Marjorie Prevost to Sanger, Feb. 15, 1932, and Sanger to Prevost, Feb. 17, 1932 [MSP-S 6:810 and MSP-L 32:225]).

24. Mary Compton Johnson to MS, Mar. 27, 1942, with Sanger's comments written in margins and on the reverse (MSP-S 20:918).

25. BCCRB Progress Report, June 1933 (MSP-L 34:683); BCCRB Doctor's Meeting, Apr. 17, 1934, and BCCRB Staff Meeting, Mar. 14, 1935 (MSP-S 61:344–46).

26. Robinson, *Seventy Birth Control Clinics*, 69–71.

27. In 1935, BCCRB physician Marie Warner argued that the women taking part in

contraceptive studies had to understand the chances of failure, and suggested that the BCCRB work with a gynecology clinic to secure therapeutic abortions for those who became pregnant during the trials. No other discussions on the issue were found (see Sanger to Prevost, Mar. 8, 1932, BCCRB Progress Report, June 1935, and Warner, "Research Recommendations").

28. Emma Hensley to Sanger, Feb. 13, 1936 (MSP-L 83:421).

29. The note, penned by Sanger's secretary Florence Rose, is somewhat ambiguous. Hensley's letter covered other topics, ranging from being treated "like a servant" by the clinic board to being forbidden to have a roommate because she feared sleeping alone at the clinic at night (Hensley to Sanger, Feb. 13, 1936 [MSP-L 83:421]).

30. For a list of medical indications, see BCCRB, *How to Establish a Birth Control Clinic* (New York: BCCRB, 1938).

31. Hannah Mayer Stone testimony before New York State Assembly, Committee on Codes, reprinted as "An Appeal to Reason," *BCR* 7:5 (May 1925): 146.

32. Ruth Topping, Memo to Bureau of Social Hygiene, Mar. 27, 1931 (BSHR).

33. Committee on Maternal Health report, ca. 1923–24 (Meyer); Leung, "'Better Babies,'" 119–21; also see MS, *Motherhood in Bondage*, chapter 15, "The Doctor Warns—But Does Not Tell," for examples of letters.

34. These statistics are drawn from ten clinics that reported patient reasons for attending, between 1927 and 1939. These clinics were: Detroit's Woman's Hospital (1931) and Harper Hospital (1931), St. Louis's Holy Cross Dispensary, Kingdom House Settlement, and Delmar Boulevard Clinic (1936), the IBCL's Chicago Medical Centers One (1927) and Five (1936), CMHA Euclid Street Clinic and West Side Branch (1936), and the Indianapolis Maternal Health Clinic (1934–35, 1938).

35. Some clinics, such as the Little Rock clinics, did set an income limit, while others, such as the St. Louis Maternal Health Clinic, used a combination of income and family size to determine eligibility on a case-by-case basis (Leung, "'Better Babies,'" 99; Statement of Clinic Policies, May 1938 [PPASLR]).

36. In a critical letter to British doctor Maurice Newfield, Eric Matsner, the medical director of the ABCL, claimed that many members of the medical profession distrusted Sanger's clinic because they feared it took patients away from private doctors. The Indianapolis Maternal Health Clinic's medical director, A. S. Johnson, agreed, reporting after a 1938 visit to the BCCRB that Sanger treated "too many pay patients" (Matsner to Newfield, May 21, 1937 [PPFAR]; Indiana Maternal Health League, Minutes, Nov. 12, 1938 [PPCIR]).

37. M. Frances Warren to Sanger, Nov. 28, 1931; Sanger, "Policies by MS," June 24, 1932 (MSP-L 32–455); Effie Lyon to Mrs. Ralph Coghlan, Apr. 25, 1934, and IBCL Annual Report, 1937–38 (PPASLR).

38. For Ryan's full testimony, see *Birth Control: Hearings before the Committee of Ways and Means, House of Representatives, 72d Congress, 1st. sess. on H.R. 11082* (Washington, D.C.: GPO, 1932). For more patient descriptions, see Mary Hughston, "Notes on the Mothers' Clinic," July 11, 1935 (MSP-L 83:564–83).

39. See Bocker, *Birth Control Methods*, 4–5, who found that 66 percent of the BCCRB patients had already tried contraceptives; Kopp, *Birth Control in Practice*,

133, found this was true for 93 percent of BCCRB patients; in "Little Rock Birth Control Clinic," *JOC* 1:10 (Oct. 1936): 173, the number was 80 percent; and Robishaw, "Study of 4,000 Patients," 430, found that 85 percent of CMHA patients has used them previously.

40. Mary M. White, "The First Impression," *National Clinic Courier*, vol. 1 (Jan. 1936): 3.

41. See Sigrid H. Brestwell, "Duties of the Desk Nurse," Apr. 18, 1929 (MSP-L 33:742B). Hilda Cornish Coates, the daughter of the Little Rock clinic founder, called herself a nurse and served as a physician's assistant, though she had no medical training (Leung, "'Better Babies,'" 80).

42. For a BCCRB patient form from 1925, see MSP-L 32:57; for the ABCL's suggested form, see "How to Start a Contraceptive Center," ca. 1936–37 (PPFAR); Robinson, *Seventy Birth Control Clinics*, 43.

43. Florence Revelle to Sanger, Sept. 28, 1931 (MSP-L 29:373B).

44. Among the clinics that offered sex education lectures were: the Montclair Maternal Health Committee (N.J.), the CMHA, the BCCRB (especially its Harlem Branch), and the clinics of the Michigan Maternal Health League. Perhaps the most extensive program was set up by Dr. Rachelle Yarros at the IBCL, where as early as 1920, 73,388 women attended 666 lectures offered over the course of a year (*Bulletin of the N.J. Birth Control League*, 1937, and CMHA Annual Report, 1935–36 [PPASLR]; Florence Rose to Marian Pascal, Jan. 31, 1936 [MSP-L 9:976–77]; Pope, "Story of Birth Control in Michigan"; Haslett, "Hull House," 270).

45. Reed, "Interview with Elizabeth Arnold," 38. Arnold supervised the clinic in the 1950s.

46. While most clinics offered a full physical examination regularly, there is evidence that some only offered a gynecological examination (Helen Buss to Janet Whitenack, May 31, 1934 [PPASLR]; Robinson, *Seventy Birth Control Clinics*, 47; Lamport, "Recreation Rooms").

47. Stix and Notestein, *Controlled Fertility*, 94, 97, 102; Robishaw, "Study of 4,000 Patients," 431.

48. Robishaw, "Study of 4,000 Patients," 426–34; Hannah Stone, "U.S.A.," in *International Medical Group for the Investigation of Contraception*, Fifth Issue (London: National Birth Control Association, 1934), 10.

49. Elizabeth Arnold contended that most private physicians did a poor job instructing their patients in contraceptives. "The patient who went to a private doctor would call the Bureau and say, 'He told me to use a diaphragm, now I don't know how to take it out. How do you take it out, I can't get it out.' And I tried to tell them on the phone or tell them to come in and just show them" (Reed, "Interview with Elizabeth Arnold," 88).

50. Robinson, *Seventy Birth Control Clinics*, 53–55; "Clinic Reports: Recreation Rooms and Settlement Birth Control Clinic, New York City," *JOC* 2:8–9 (Aug.–Sept. 1937): 164; ABCL, "How to Start a Contraceptive Center," ca. 1936–37 (PPFAR).

51. Leung, "'Better Babies,'" 165–67; "Increasing Clinic Attendance," *National Clinic Courier* 2:1 (Jan. 1936): 1–2 [Dennett 16:466–68]; Robinson, *Seventy Birth*

Control Clinics, 53–55; "Clinic Reports: Recreation Rooms," 164; and ABCL, "How to Start a Contraceptive Center," ca. 1936–37 (PPFAR).

52. For more on infertility, see David Loth and John Rock, *Voluntary Parenthood* (New York: Random House, 1949), and Margaret S. Marsh, *The Empty Cradle: Infertility in America from Colonial Times to the Present* (Baltimore: Johns Hopkins University Press, 1996); for the PPFA's program, see PPFA, "Suggested Policy on Our Responsibility for the Positive Aspects of Planned Parenthood and Suggestions for Action," Apr. 6, 1943 (MSP-S 65:190).

53. Tone's *Devices and Desires* has the best coverage of contraceptive technology in the 1920s and 1930s; Robert Dickinson, "Editorial: Impressions of the Recent Conference on Contraceptive Research and Clinical Practice" *JOC* 2:1 (Jan. 1937): 12.

54. Stone, "Notes on a Roundtable Discussion."

55. Some clinic activists agreed that intelligent women were more likely to be able to use the clinic successfully (Raymond Pearl, "Contraception and Fertility in 2,000 Women," *Human Biology* 4:3 [Sept. 1932]: 363–408; Stone, "Notes on a Roundtable Discussion"; Nash, "Planned Parenthood," 128–29 [quote]).

56. See Bocker, *Birth Control Methods,* 9–11; Warner, "Research Recommendations"; Helen Holt, "A Summary of Research on the Spermicidal Powers of Contraceptives in the U.S.A.," Dec. 30, 1933 (MSP-L 30:176); Stone, "Notes on a Roundtable Discussion."

57. Lydia deVilbiss, "Preliminary Report on the Use of Foam Powder and Rubber Sponge Pessary in the White and Colored Clinics," Nov. 30, 1936, and deVilbiss to Eric Matsner, Jan. 4, 1936 (PPFAR); H. M. Carleton, "Reports on Pathological Tests of Two Samples of Foam Powder and One of Foam Jelly," Aug. 27 and Sept. 9, 1936, and Feb. 15, 1937 (MSP-S 15:577).

58. Meyer, *Any Friend,* 150–53, 159.

59. Bocker, *Birth Control Methods,* 9.

60. Meyer, *Any Friend,* 152; Warner, "Research Recommendations."

61. Higley, "Clinic Reports: Men's Consultation Service" (quote 1); BCCRB, "Questions Relating to the Work of the Birth Control Clinical Research Bureau," 1933 (MSP-L 33:576); Hannah Stone, "Birth Control as a Factor in the Sex Life of a Woman," in Norman Haire, ed., *Proceedings of the Third Congress of the World League for Sexual Reform* (London: Kegan Paul, 1930), 156 (quotes 2–4); Rachelle S. Yarros, "Birth Control and Sex Hygiene," *BCR* 6:7 (July 1924): 202 (quote 5).

62. Robinson, *Seventy Birth Control Clinics,* 31. For evidence of these services after 1939, see Guttmacher, *Planned Parenthood Beginnings,* 18, 27, 115, and 142; and Mrs. V. L. Board, Thomas Cunningham, Imogene Genter, and Mrs. Charles Kessler, "Denver Celebrates Silver Anniversary," 1951 (PPFAR).

63. Sanger to Alfred H. Tyrer, Feb. 23, 1932 (MSP-L 32:110).

64. Robinson, *Seventy Birth Control Clinics,* 150–52; Norman Haire, "Sterilization of the Unfit," paper given at the First American Birth Control Conference, Nov. 1921, published in *BCR* 6:2 (Feb. 1922): 10–11.

65. IBCL, "Report on Birth Control Conference Held at the Chicago Woman's Aid Society," Dec. 5, 1929 (CWASR); Los Angeles Mothers' Clinic, "Suggestions."

For more on the desire of patients for sterilization over contraception, see Schoen, *Choice and Coercion*, 77–80.

66. In her promotional literature, deVilbiss quoted a Johns Hopkins University study that found that 39 percent of whites and 70 percent of African Americans were "feebleminded" and thus candidates for sterilization. She claimed to have waiting lists for vasectomies and had to refer overflow cases to city and county hospitals (Lydia deVilbiss, "Clinical Experiences with Vasectomy," *JOC* 3:10 [Oct. 1937]: 173–75; deVilbiss, "Outline Plan of Organization for Mothers' Health Clubs," ca. 1933 [quote], Miami Mothers' Health Clinic, "Relief or Cure" 1935, and deVilbiss to Catherine Bangs, ca. 1934 [PPFAR]).

67. See Palama Settlement Mothers' Health Clinic Report, 1937 (quote 3), and Extract from a Letter from a Member of the Executive Committee of the Mass. Birth Control League, Mar. 22, 1935 (quotes 1–2; PPFAR). Neither the personal papers of either deVilbiss or Cass, nor the records of their clinics, have been found.

CHAPTER 3: CLINIC ACTIVISTS

1. Gordon's observations and analysis, repeated in her 2002 update *Moral Right* (171–210), were challenged by Meyer in "Birth Control Policy," 235 and 270, and in Leung, "'Better Babies,'" 211–14. McCann stretches Gordon's argument further by claiming a divide between the male-focused BCFA and the woman-focused "Sangerists," but her analysis is also focused on national leagues (McCann, *Birth Control Politics*, 176–77, 185, and 190).

2. John Price Jones, *Report on the ABCL*, 62 and 95 (MSP-L 27:685 and 701); Arthur W. Packard's recommendations on funding the NCFLBC, 1934–37 (OMRR), and Penelope Huse to Sanger, Jan. 15, 1937 (MSP-S 14:214).

3. Caroline Robinson, "How Shall We Start a Clinic?" *BCR* 16:5 (May 1932): 143–44.

4. Holz, "Birth Control Clinic in America," 42–43; Sanger to Lawrence Dunham, July 31, 1928 (MSP-L 35:161).

5. See Jeanette C. Small, "Report of the Maine Birth Control League to ABCL," ca. Jan. 1934 (PPFAR); Buffalo Family Relations Institute Annual Report, 1937–38; Minnesota Birth Control League Annual Report, 1932–33; and Hartford Maternal Health Clinic Annual Report, 1937–38 (PPASLR); John Price Jones Corporation, "Survey and Plan of Fund-Raising for the BCCRB and the NCFLBC," Sept. 15, 1930 (MSP-S 61:476).

6. Gamble to Donald West, Jan. 9 1934 (Gamble); Holz, "Birth Control Clinic in America," 58; Clara Worthington, "Annual Reports of the State Member Leagues for 1936 to the ABCL, Birth Control League of Delaware," and Syracuse Maternal Health Clinic, Annual Report, 1939 (PPFAR); Leung, "'Better Babies,'" 163, and 75–76; Hartford Maternal Health Clinic, 1937–38 Report and CMHA Annual Report, 1935–36 (PPASLR); Report of Birth Control Work of the Recreation Rooms and Settlement Branch Birth Control Clinic Maternal Health Center, Mar. 1935 (MSP-L 32:312–14A).

7. Sanger, *My Fight*, 191.

8. Nelson to Sanger, May 7, 1929 (MSP-L 85:265).

9. See the state-by-state appendices in Vreeland's, "Process of Reform," for pre–World War I birth control organizing.

10. Among the ABCL board members in the 1920s were: Katharine Beach Day (1853–1942), Annie Goodrich Porritt (1861–1932), Charlotte Hoffman Delafield (1865–1947), May Merrill Billings (1874–1965), Frances Brooks Ackermann (1875–1935), Ida Haar Timme (1875–1940), Juliet Barrett Rublee (1875–1966), Mabel Whitney Blagden (1875–1968), Margaret Sanger (1879–1966), and Eleanor Dwight Jones (1880–1965). Dates for activists come from the U.S. Census and Social Security Death Index.

11. "Mrs. Lewis Delafield," *New York Times*, Apr. 25, 1947; Sanger, *Autobiography*, 230 (quote).

12. "Obituaries," *Winnetka Talk*, June 28, 1945.

13. "Death Takes Mrs. Nelson," *Reading Eagle*, July 11, 1940; Mary Nelson to Sanger, Mar. 8, 1934 (MSP-L 103:690B) (quote).

14. For some of Sanger's speeches in these years, see "Woman and Birth Control," 1916 (MSP-L 129:12), "Breaking into the South—A Contrast," *BCR* 2:12 (Dec. 1919): 7–8 (MSP-S 70:829), and "Address to Pennsylvania Birth Control League," Feb. 27, 1929 (MSP-L 128:446).

15. Some of the clinics supported by Junior League women included the Birmingham Alabama Maternal Health Clinic, the University Hospital Maternal Health Clinic in Augusta, Georgia, the Pasadena Woman's Hospital Clinic in California, and the Little Rock and Cleveland clinics (Guttmacher, *Planned Parenthood Beginnings*, 12–13, 37; Donald West to Clarence Gamble, Oct. 24, 1933 [Gamble]; Leung, "'Better Babies,'" 78, 86–87, 95; Meyer, *Any Friend*, 127).

16. Leung, "'Better Babies,'" 26–29, 77–80.

17. Ibid., 83–89, 43, 90, 95.

18. Edna Brush Perkins was the daughter of Charles Brush Sr., Dorothy Brush's father-in-law. Rosalyn Weir was his grand-niece. An active social reformer, Perkins worked for suffrage, founded the Woman's City Club, and was active in the Anti-Tuberculosis League and the Welfare Foundation of Cleveland (Meyer, *Any Friend*, 65–69; "Edna Brush Perkins," in *The Encyclopedia of Cleveland History*, http://ech.cwru.edu, accessed Sept. 11, 2009).

19. The quote is by Elizabeth Grew Bacon, from Madeline Gray, *Margaret Sanger* (New York: R. Marek, 1979), 145–46.

20. Katz, *Selected Papers* 2:469–71.

21. Sanger to Lydia deVilbiss, Jan. 18, 1935 (MSP-L 8:282).

22. Anna S. McHugh, "Nebraska Maternal Health Association Annual Report to the American Birth Control League," 1936 (PPASLR).

23. Meyer, *Any Friend*, 58–61; see also the Indiana Maternal Health League Board of Directors, Minutes, Oct. 8, 1934 (PPCIR). For details on the Town Hall Raid, see Katz, *Selected Papers* 1:328–31.

24. Leung, "'Better Babies,'" 128.

25. McCann, *Birth Control Politics*, 99–100.

26. Caroline Jean Acker, "Pearl, Raymond," http://www.anb.org/articles/13/13-01279

.html, Diane B. Paul, "East, Edward Murray," http://www.anb.org/articles/13/13-00461 .htm, and Karen Rader, "Little, Clarence Cook," http://www.anb.org/articles/13/13-02444.html, in *American National Biography Online*, Feb. 2000; McCann, *Birth Control Politics*, 121; Pearl, "Contraception and Fertility in 2,000 Women," and "Contraception and Fertility in 4,945 Married Women: A Second Report on a Study of Family Limitation," *Human Biology* (May 1934): 355–401.

27. The best examples of these are Henry Goddard's ubiquitous *The Kallikak Family* (New York: Macmillan, 1912), and Arthur Estabrook's *The Jukes in 1915* (Washington, D.C.: Carnegie Institute, 1915). See McCann, *Birth Control Politics*, 99–134, for a detailed treatment of eugenics and birth control.

28. In the 1930s, the ABCL and the American Eugenics Association considered merging, but could not find common ground (McCann, *Birth Control Politics*, 180–81). For more on women eugenicists, see Edward Larson, "'In the Finest, Most Womanly Way': Women in the Southern Eugenics Movement," *American Journal of Legal History* 39:2 (Apr. 1995): 120–22, 139–40; Kevles, *In the Name of Eugenics*, 64.

29. "William Hazlett Upson Dies, Wrote Alexander Botts Series," *New York Times*, Feb. 8, 1975; Upson, "Letter to the Future," 1936 (Upson).

30. 1930 U.S. Census; Charles Stephan, "The Unitarian Church of Lincoln," *Bring O Past Your Honor*, Mar. 1986; *Nebraska State Journal*, Jan. 9, 1940; Nebraska State Historical Society Library Photograph Collection.

31. Sarah Lawrence's study of grassroots African American birth control in the South posits that networks of lay women and nurses provided contraceptives to rural African American women, but her treatment of the Negro Project and the BCFA efforts and motives lacks nuance and detail (Lawrence, "On Their Own Terms: African Americans and Birth Control in the Rural South, 1900–1942," Ph.D. diss., Pennsylvania State University, 2007).

32. For African American activism in general, see Paula Giddings, *When and Where I Enter: The Impact of Black Women on Race and Sex in America* (New York: Morrow, 1984), and Darline Clark Hine, *Black Women in White* (Bloomington: Indiana University Press, 1992). The African Americans most often quoted on birth control, W. E. B. Du Bois, W. G. Alexander, and Marcus Garvey, are all better known as civil rights activists, not as birth control activists (see Roberts, *Killing the Black Body*, 82–88; McCann, *Birth Control Politics*, 142–44; Hart, "Who Should Have the Children?" 71–84).

33. Alexander, "Medical Viewpoint," 175.

34. Rodrique, "Afro-American Community," 135–36.

35. Kopp, *Birth Control in Practice*, 49.

36. The advisory council included doctors, most associated with Harlem Hospital: Lucien Brown, May Chinn (1896–1980), Harold L. Ellis (1895–1989), Alonzo DeGrate Smith (1890–1970), James L. Wilson, and Louis T. Wright (1891–1952); nurses Marion Hernandez, Mabel Keaton Staupers (1890–1989), and Jane Ryder Fisher (1894-?); clergymen Horatio Hill and William Lloyd Imes; teachers Lois Allen, Bessye Bearden (1883–1943), and white philanthropist Caroline Bamberger Fuld (1864–1944).

37. Rodrique, "Afro-American Community," 135–46.

38. The three lay advisory council members all held jobs—Lois Allen worked for the Urban League, Bessye Bearden was a journalist, businesswoman, civic leader, and mother of Romaire Bearden; Jane Ryder Fisher was a high school teacher married to prominent Harlem Renaissance writer and physician Rudolph Fisher (Darryl Lyman, *Great African American Women* [Middle Village, N.Y.: J. David, 2005], 275; Venetria K Patton and Maureen Honey, eds., *Double-Take: A Revisionist Harlem Renaissance Anthology* [New Brunswick, N.J.: Rutgers University Press, 2001], 386).

39. BCCRB, "Tentative Plans for Proposed Birth Control Clinic at the N.Y. Urban League," Mar. 10, 1933, and Mabel Staupers to MS, Mar. 13, 1935 (MSP-L 33:339 and 83A).

40. Harlem Advisory Council Minutes, Sept. 23, Nov. 5, 1931, Mar. 23, Oct. 25, 1932, Jan. 25 and Mar. 31, 1933, BCCRB, "Suggestions Approved by Mrs. Sanger, New Program for Harlem Branch," Oct. 18, 1932, Harlem Branch Statistical Report, Feb. 1, 1930 to Dec. 31, 1930, and Florence Rose to Marian Pascal, Jan. 31, 1936 (MSP-L 33:178–86, MSP-S 61:462, and MSP-L 9:976); Granger, "Birth Control in Harlem," 91–92.

41. Hazel Zborowski, "Resume of Meeting Held at 515 Madison Avenue, May 28, 1935" (MSP-L 33:350).

42. W. Michael Byrd and Linda A. Clayton, *An American Health Dilemma: Race, Medicine, and Health Care in the United States, 1900–2000*, vol. 2 (New York: Routledge, 2002), 174–83.

43. Robert G. Weisbord, *Genocide? Birth Control and the Black American* (Westport, Conn.: Greenwood Press, 1975), 43.

44. Rodrique, "Afro-American Community," 90, 182; McCann, *Birth Control Politics*, 145–47; Hart, "Who Should Have the Children?" 71–84, and "African Americans, Health Care, and the Reproductive Freedom Movement in Detroit, 1918–1945," Ph.D. diss., University of Michigan (1998); Roberts, *Killing the Black Body*, 82–84; McCann, *Birth Control Politics*, 148–53.

45. See Bousfield, "Negro Public Health Work Needs Birth Control," 170–71.

46. Giddings, *When and Where I Enter*, 97–98.

47. Staupers to Sanger, Aug. 2, 1935 (MSP-L 33:84).

48. Ferebee, "Planned Parenthood," 9.

49. No accurate count of these clinics is known. In "Afro-American Community," Jessie Rodrique asserts that there were only two states, California and Oklahoma, with African American owned and operated clinics (179).

50. Lewis and Young, "Baltimore's Negro Maternal Health Center," 93–94; Rodrique, "Afro-American Community," 194.

51. Hazel Moore "Confidential Report," Dec. 14, 1935 (PPFAR).

52. Rodrique, "Afro-American Community," 179 n. 13, 181–82; "Dr. Ruth Temple Ends Long Career with City," *Los Angeles Times*, Dec. 13, 1962.

53. Rodrique's "Afro-American Community" offers the best descriptions of these clinics, but because she relied on scattered newspaper coverage for much of her information, she provides little depth on any one clinic.

54. S. Adolphus Knopf to Sanger, Feb. 26, 1929 (MSP-L 57:347).

55. A sampling of clinic personnel at independent clinics, taken from pamphlets, letterheads, and promotional materials, finds that of 278 medical advisors, only three were women (98.9 percent were male).

56. Regina M. Sanchez-Morantz, *Sympathy and Science: Women Physicians in American Medicine* (New York: Oxford University Press, 1985), 234, 249.

57. Chesler, "Interview with Sarah Marcus," 29.

58. James W. Reed, "Stone, Abraham, and Hannah Mayer Stone," http://www.anb.org/articles/12/12-00887.html in *American National Biography Online*, Feb. 2000, accessed Sept. 11, 2009. For some of Stone's published clinical research, see "Therapeutic Contraception," *Medical Journal and Record* 6 (Mar. 21, 1938): 612–14; "Present-Day Problems in Contraception," *JOC* 1:1 (Nov. 1935): 3–5; and "The Vaginal Diaphragm," *JOC* 3:6–7 (June–July 1938): 123–27.

59. Stone to Sanger, Mar. 27, 1932, and Cele Damon to Sanger, Mar. 1938 (quote) (MSP-L 32:369 and MSP-S 16:607).

60. Sanger, diary entry, July 14, 1941 (MSP-S 70:57–58).

61. Sanger, *Autobiography*, 360–61.

62. Chesler, "Birth Control Movement," in *Jewish Women in America: An Historical Encyclopedia, vol. 1*, ed. Paula Hyman and Deborah Dash Moore (New York: Routledge, 1997). Other prominent Jewish birth control clinicians were Bessie Moses, Lena Levine, and Nadina Kavinoky.

63. See Yarros, "Birth Control and Sex Hygiene," 199–203; "Birth Control and Its Relation to Health and Welfare," *Medical Woman's Journal* 32 (1925): 261–64; and "The Future of the Birth Control Clinic," *BCR* 16:11 (Nov. 1932): 262–68.

64. Chesler, "Sarah Marcus Interview," 12–19 and 34–36 (quotes 1–2); Meyer, "Birth Control Policy," 80; *Encyclopedia of Cleveland History*, http://ech.cwru.edu, accessed Sept. 11, 2009.

65. It was not until the 1950s that Rauschkolb was granted privileges at two Cleveland hospitals (*Encyclopedia of Cleveland History*, http://ech.cwru.edu, accessed Sept. 11, 2009).

66. Stone, "Notes on a Roundtable Discussion."

67. "Dr. Elizabeth Pissoort," *New York Times*, Dec. 5, 1958.

68. Leung, "'Better Babies,'" 125.

69. BCCRB summary, June 1937 (PPFAR).

70. S. Adolphus Knopf to Sanger, Feb. 26, 1929 (MSP-L 57:347).

71. "Dr. A. N. Creadick, Taught at Yale, 72," *New York Times*, July 25, 1956; 1930 Census; Indiana Maternal Health League, Board of Directors Emergency Meeting, July 6, 1939 (PPCIR).

72. Garrow, *Liberty and Sexuality*, 57, 82, 731 n. 95.

73. Clarence Gamble to Donald West, June 15, 1933 (Gamble).

74. Robinson, *Seventy Birth Control Clinics*, 123; telephone conversation with Mount Sinai Hospital archivist, Barbara Niss, Feb. 1, 2000.

75. Settlement house clinics were responsible for twenty-one of the fifty-nine female members of medical advisory boards and the remaining thirty-nine were hired by independent clinics.

76. Exceptions were Dr. Alvan J. Goodbar and Dr. Robert Crossen, who were also presidents of the Missouri Maternal Health Association. After Goodbar's tenure was up, the association selected a woman, Helen W. McPheeters, to head the clinic until the end of the 1930s (Missouri Maternal Health Association minutes, Mar. 20, 1933 [PPASLR]).

77. The Medical Society held that it was unethical for the clinic to refer women to private physicians, despite the fact that they permitted other city agencies to do so (Helen S. Buss to Richard N. Pierson, Oct. 3, 1939 [PPASLR]).

78. Gladys Gaylord, "Several Aspects of Public Acceptance," Annual Meeting of the Pennsylvania Birth Control Federation, Nov. 28, 1939 (PPFAR).

79. Stone to Sanger, Mar. 27, 1932 (MSP-L 32:369).

80. Sanger to Marjorie Prevost, Jan. 27, 1932 (MSP-L 32:213–15).

81. Chesler, "Sarah Marcus Interview," 28; Sanger to Marjorie Prevost, Jan. 27, 1932, and Sanger to Hannah Stone, June 26, 1929 (quote) (MSP-L 32:213 and MSP-S 5:132). Kelman went on to work at the ABCL clinic at Stuyvesant House.

82. The CMHA went furthest to try to attract male support, sponsoring special informational "men's luncheons" for the heads of social agencies. In 1938, the ABCL focused their fund-raising towards attracting more support from male donors. Their reported successes underscore the feminized nature of birth control support—that year they raised $151,000, only $33,000 of which came from these new efforts (Meyer, *Any Friend,* 108–11; ABCL Annual Report, 1938 [PPFAR]).

83. See Eric Matsner, "Annual Report of the ABCL Medical Department for 1937" (PPFAR).

84. For the academy's findings, see James Alexander Miller to Sanger, Apr. 4, 1930 (MSP-L 65:430).

85. Gladys Gaylord, "Several Aspects of Acceptance," speech to the Pennsylvania Birth Control Federation annual meeting, Nov. 28, 1939 (quote) (PPASLR); Gaylord, "Men and a Maternal Health Program," 103–4.

86. Eleanor Dwight Jones was a Radcliffe graduate who married Frederick Robertson Jones, an economist and insurance expert. A supporter of women's suffrage, Jones worked as a teacher and was active in the Municipal League, the Woman's City Club, the Cosmopolitan Club, and the League of Women Voters. Jones listed "eugenics" as one of her hobbies (Durward Howes, ed., *American Women, 1935–1940: A Composite Biographical Dictionary* [Detroit: Gale Research, 1981]; *Radcliffe College Class of 1902 Secretary's Fifth Report,* June 1927, 59).

87. Catherine Clement Bangs, the wife of lawyer Francis N. Bangs, claimed to have been inspired by Sanger's 1921 Town Hall address. She was also involved in Everybody's Thrift Shop, an enterprise sponsored by sixteen New York charities, and was a member of the Cosmopolitan Club ("Mrs. Bangs, Leader in Birth Control," *New York Times,* July 25, 1966).

88. Clarence Cook Little (1888–1971) was a Harvard-trained geneticist, cancer expert, and educator, not a physician. He briefly served as assistant director of the Carnegie Institution's State for Experimental Evolution under eugenicist Charles Davenport, but left to become president of the University of Michigan. In 1929

Little was fired over his forward-thinking advice to students, including his support for birth control ("Dr. Clarence Little, Cancer Researcher, Dies at 83," *New York Times*, Dec. 23, 1971.

89. Pierson had formerly served on the Medical Advisory Board of the New York Committee of Mother's Health Centers, but was not active in the movement before 1939 (*Who Was Who*, vol. 7, 1971–80 [Chicago: Marquis, 1981], 455).

90. Morris had worked with the Baltimore City Public Health Department and the Delaware Public Health Department, and had worked in hospitals in Detroit and Baltimore (BCFA Citizens' Committee for Planned Parenthood, press release, Apr. 10, 1939 [PPFAR]).

91. The vice presidents were: Drs. Robert L. Dickinson, Frederick C. Holden, Clarence Cook Little, and sociologist Henry Pratt Fairchild, most holdovers from the ABCL board ("Birth Control Rift Ended by Merger," *New York Times*, Jan. 19, 1939).

92. Lay women ran the BCCRB until the merger, though its advisory board was staffed by professional men. Among those frustrated by their demotions were stalwarts like Florence Rose (1903–69), who had held a variety of secretarial and administrative posts for the BCCRB and NCFLBC. She resigned in 1943. Cele Armstrong Damon, the BCCRB's executive secretary, resigned from the BCFA in 1941 to return to the BCCRB. Marguerite Benson, the executive director of the ABCL, was another casualty of the merger, resigning in July 1939 (Finding aid to the Florence Rose Papers, Smith College; Damon to Sanger, Apr. 20, 1939, and Apr. 1, 1941 [MSP-S 16:709, S19:124]; Williams, *Every Child a Wanted Child*, 285).

93. Eric Matsner, "Annual Report of the ABCL Medical Department for 1937" (PPFAR).

94. BCFA Annual Report, 1939 (MSP-S 63:373).

95. Arkansas Eugenics Association, 1931–33 report, 1931–34 report, 1935 report, "Your Community and Birth Control," 1937 and 1938 reports. The association's treasurer was Charles H. Wickard Jr. (1886-?), who was in sales (AEAR; 1920 Census).

96. The first president of the IBCL was Professor James A. Field of the University of Chicago, but after his death in 1927 women held all offices (IBCL Annual Report, 1937–38).

97. IBCL Annual Reports, 1925–39.

CHAPTER 4: EUGENICS AND RACE AT THE CLINIC

1. See Charles Davenport, *Heredity in Relation to Eugenics* (New York: H. Holt and Co., 1911); Kevles, *In the Name of Eugenics*, 44–54; and McCann, *Birth Control Politics*, 104–6.

2. There is an extensive historiography on eugenics, but most of these works deal only tangentially with the birth control movement. See in particular, Kevles, *In the Name of Eugenics;* Wendy Kline, *Building a Better Race: Gender, Sexuality, and Eugenics from the Turn of the Century to the Baby Boom* (Berkeley: University of California Press, 2001); Steven Selden, *Inheriting Shame: The Story of Eugenics and Racism in America* (New York: Teachers College Press, 1999). McCann's *Birth Control Policy*, 99–134, offers the most detailed analysis.

3. For the "mainline" and "reform" categories, see Kevles, *In the Name of Eugenics*, 88, 173–75.

4. See Lothrop Stoddard, *The Rising Tide of Color* (New York: Charles Scribner's Sons, 1921); Madison Grant, *The Passing of the Great Race* (New York: Scribner, 1916); Kevles, *In the Name of Eugenics*, 46–47, 75; McCann, *Birth Control Politics*, 117.

5. For Du Bois's views on birth control, including his contention that better-off Negro families ought to have more children than those who had less economic means, see his "Opinion," *Crisis* 24 (Oct. 1922): 248.

6. Paul Popenoe was one such critic, who argued that birth control resulted in racial degeneration because it was more widely used among the better classes (McCann, *Birth Control Policy*, 108).

7. Leung, "'Better Babies,'" 36, quoting Rabbi Ira E. Saunders, in a 1978 interview by Charlotte Gadbury.

8. McCann, *Birth Control Politics*, 120–21; Gaylord, "The Eugenic Value of a Maternal Health Center," JOC 3:3 (Mar. 1938): 51–53; Leung, "'Better Babies,'" 46; and Robinson, *Seventy Birth Control Clinics*, 152. For links between the ABCL and the American Eugenics Society, see Franks, *Margaret Sanger's Eugenic Legacy*, 76–77.

9. For general background on reforms, see Meckel, *Save the Babies*, and Kathleen D. McCarthy, *Lady Bountiful Revisited: Women, Philanthropy, and Power* (New Brunswick, N.J.: Rutgers University Press, 1990).

10. U.S. House of Representatives, *Birth Control Hearings before the Committee on the Judiciary, House of Representatives*, 72d. Congress, 2d sess., on H.R. 5978, Jan. 18, 19, 1934 (Washington, D.C.: GPO, 1934), 151–54.

11. McCann, *Birth Control Politics*, 19; Claire M. Roche, "Reproducing the Working Class: Tillie Olson, Margaret Sanger, and American Eugenics," in *Evolution and Eugenics in American Literature, 1880–1940*, ed. Lois A. Cuddy and Claire Roche (Lewisburg, Penn.: Bucknell University Press, 2003), 259–75; see also Chesler, "Afterword" in *Woman of Valor*, rev. ed. (New York: Simon and Schuster, 2007), 484.

12. For examples, see Franks, *Margaret Sanger's Eugenic Legacy*, and Marlene Garber Fried, *From Abortion to Reproductive Freedom: Transforming a Movement* (Boston: South End Press, 1990), 20–21.

13. Sanger, *Family Limitation*, 3.

14. Sanger, "Birth Control and Racial Betterment," *BCR* 3:2 (Feb. 1919): 11–12.

15. Sanger, *Woman and the New Race*, 35–37.

16. Sanger, "Testimony on N.Y.S. Assembly Bill," Apr. 10, 1923, in Katz, *Selected Papers* 1:360–65.

17. Sanger, "My Way to Peace," Jan. 17, 1932, and "Statement of the Southern Tour," Nov. 12, 1938 (MSP-L 130:198 and 754).

18. Sanger to Sidney L. Lasell Jr., Feb. 13, 1934 (MSP-S 8:541–42).

19. Sanger, *Pivot of Civilization*, 171, 175.

20. William Hazlett Upson, "Letter to the Future, 1936" (Upson).

21. William H. Schneider, "Toward the Improvement of the Race: The History of Eugenics in France," *Journal of Modern History* 54:2 (June 1982): 268–91; Lara

Marks, *Women and Children First: International Maternal and Infant Welfare, 1870–1945* (London: Routledge, 1982).

22. Sanger, *Pivot of Civilization,* 168.

23. The only two infertility programs begun before 1939 were offered at Cincinnati's Maternal Health Committee Downtown Clinic and Chicago's Mandel Clinic, both based in hospitals. For the Dickinson incident, see NCMH, "Report," ca. 1923–24 (Meyer); see also Robinson, *Seventy Birth Control Clinics,* 31–32; Guttmacher, *Planned Parenthood Beginnings;* and Thomas B. Turner, *Heritage of Excellence: The Johns Hopkins Medical Institutions, 1914–1947* (Baltimore: Johns Hopkins University Press, 1974), 400.

24. Ian Robert Dowbiggan, *Keeping America Sane: Psychiatry and Eugenics in the United States and Canada, 1880–1940* (Ithaca, N.Y.: Cornell University Press, 2003), 191–230; Paul Popenoe and Roswell Johnson, *Applied Eugenics* (New York: Macmillan, 1920), 197–98; Stephen Jay Gould, "Carrie Buck's Daughter," in *The Flamingo's Smile: Reflections in Natural History* (New York: Norton, 1985), 307–13.

25. He claimed that after his wife secretly started using birth control she had two still births and then a hysterectomy (Raymond Magee to Sanger, Apr. 11, 1935 [MSP-L 9:375]).

26. In proportion to the general population, American birth control clinics reached more middle class and skilled laborers as patients, while British clinics had higher numbers of the very poor (Robinson, *Seventy Birth Control Clinics,* 89).

27. Mary Hughston, "Notes on the Mothers' Clinic," July 11, 1935 (MSP-L 83:564).

28. Sanger to Alfred H. Tyrer, Feb. 23, 1932 (MSP-L 12:110).

29. Kline, *Building a Better Race,* 49.

30. Sanger, *Pivot of Civilization,* 169.

31. Eric Matsner, "Statement Approved by the Executive Committee of the National Medical Council on Birth Control," Oct. 28, 1937, included in the 1937 ABCL Annual Report (PPFAR); see also Robinson, *Seventy Birth Control Clinics,* 102–3, and McCann, *Birth Control Politics,* 108–9.

32. Robinson, *Seventy Birth Control Clinics,* 102.

33. Holz, "Birth Control Clinic in America," 43–45; Leung, "'Better Babies,'" 164; Kopp, *Birth Control in Practice,* 37.

34. Mary Hughston, "Profiles of Tucson Mothers' Clinic Patients," July 11–25, 1935 (MSP-LC 83:564–83); the photos of the families were not found.

35. Client to Sanger, July 5, 1932 (MSP-S 7:218).

36. See Hart, "Homes of the Poor," 319–20; "An Experiment in Constructive Family Help, Part I," *BCR* 11:3 (Mar. 1927): 71–72, 78; Condit, "Underprivileged."

37. Seibels, "Integration of Pregnancy Spacing"; Robinson, *Seventy Birth Control Clinics,* 152.

38. The Baltimore Bureau for Contraceptive Advice estimated that only 1 percent of their cases (which all had some medical component) were "eugenic" in nature (Robinson, *Seventy Birth Control Clinics,* 153).

39. Lydia deVilbiss, "Outline Plan of Organization for Mothers' Health Clubs," ca. 1933 (PPFAR).

40. Haslett, "Hull House," 267.

41. Mary Hughston, "Notes on the Mothers' Clinic," July 11, 1935 (MSP-L 83:564–83).

42. Hart, "Homes of the Poor," 319–20.

43. Dickinson and Morris, "Birth Control Centers," 591–93; Anderson, "Private Choices vs. Public Voices," 67–68; "News from the States," *BCR* 23:1 (Jan. 1939): 157; Hughston, "Notes on the Mothers' Clinic," July 11, 1935 (MSP-L 83:564–83); Tasker, "Mothers' Clinic," 251–53; extract from a Member of the Executive Committee of the Mass. Birth Control League, Mar. 22, 1935 (PPFAR).

44. Roberts, *Killing the Black Body*, 7–9; Rodrique, "Afro-American Community," 101–2.

45. Ferebee, "Planned Parenthood," 7.

46. Lewis and Young, "Baltimore's Negro Maternal Health Center," 93–94; Ohio Maternal Health Association Annual Report, Oct. 1938, and Indiana Maternal Health League Board of Directors Minutes, Oct. 8, 1934 (PPCIR); Anderson, "Private Choices vs. Public Voices," 7–8, 67.

47. Dorothy B. Atkinson, "Report of the Minnesota Birth Control League to the Annual Meeting of the ABCL," Jan. 16, 1935 (PPFAR); Rodrique, "Afro-American Community," 187 n. 23.

48. Rodrique, "Afro-American Community," 189–90.

49. Jean B. Tachau, "Annual Reports of the Kentucky Birth Control League to the American Birth Control League," 1936 (PPFAR).

50. Rodrique, "Afro-American Community," 206–8; and Hazel Moore "Confidential Report," Dec. 14, 1935 (PPFAR).

51. Sanger, *Autobiography*, 213–14.

52. Mark Haller, *Eugenics: Hereditarian Attitudes in American Thought* (New Brunswick, N.J.: Rutgers University Press, 1963), and John Higham, *Strangers in the Land: Patterns of American Nativism, 1860–1925* (New York: Atheneum, 1955).

53. Pearl gathered data on twenty-five thousand women from 1929 to 1932 in New York City, Philadelphia, Baltimore, Washington, and Chicago. He later backpedaled, concluding that African American women were no more fertile than white women and that their higher birth rates argued that they practiced birth control less frequently and "somewhat less intelligently and carefully when they do practice it" (Pearl, "Preliminary Notes on a Cooperative Investigation of Family Limitation," *Milbank Memorial Fund Quarterly* 11:1 [1933]: 37–60, and "Second Progress Report on a Study of Family Limitation," *Milbank Memorial Fund Quarterly* 12 [1934]: 248–69).

54. U.S. House of Representatives, *Birth Control Hearings on H.R. 5978;* Rodrique, "Afro-American Community," 75–76; and Roberts, *Killing the Black Body*, 84–87.

55. "Editorial," George S. Schuyler, "Quantity or Quality," and W. E. B. Du Bois, "Black Folk and Birth Control," all from *BCR* 16:6 (June 1932): 161–67; Rodrique, "Black Community," 335–36.

56. Rodrique, "Afro-American Community," 131–33; Granger, "Birth Control in Harlem," 91–92; see also Lamport, "Recreation Rooms"; Texas Birth Control League, Annual Report to the ABCL, ca. 1936 (PPFAR); and Marie Warner, "Birth Control and the Negro," in BCCRB Progress Report, June 1935 (MSP-S 61:790).

57. Chesler, "Sarah Marcus Interview," 24.

58. Leung, "'Better Babies,'" 99–100.

59. Roberts, *Killing the Black Body*, 7–9; see also Preston Valien and Alberta Price Fitzgerald, "Attitudes of the Negro Mother toward Birth Control," *American Journal of Sociology* 55 (Nov. 1949): 279–83; Rodrique, "Afro-American Community," 46–48; Missouri Maternal Health Association, Board Minutes, Sept. 27, 1935 (PPASLR).

60. DeVilbiss to Allison Pierce Moore, July 15, 1937, deVilbiss to Eric Matsner, Jan. 28, 1936; Linda Gordon, *Woman's Body, Woman's Right: A Social History of Birth Control in America* (New York: Grossman, 1976), 330 (quote).

61. Missouri Maternal Health Association, Board Minutes, Apr. 19 and Sept. 27, 1935 (PPASLR) (quote 1); Marjorie Prevost to MS, May 4, 1932, MS to Prevost, May 8, 1932 (quote 2) (MSP-L 32:264–65, 266–67); McCann, *Birth Control Politics*, 142–43.

62. Rodrique, "Black Community," 337–38; Lydia deVilbiss to Eric Matsner, Jan. 26, 1938 (PPFAR); Harlem Branch Advisory Minutes, Mar. 23, 1932, Oct. 25, 1932, and Jan. 25, 1933; Sanger to Marjorie Prevost, Feb. 2, 1932 (MSP-L 33:181–81, 32:216).

63. McCann, *Birth Control Politics*, 137–48; Hart, "Who Should Have the Children?" 71–84.

64. Harlem Advisory Council Minutes, Mar. 23 and Oct. 25, 1932, Jan. 25, 1933 (MSP-L 33:181–84); Midian Othello Bousfield to Michael Marks Davis, Apr. 9, 1932 (MSP-L 31:199); McCann, *Birth Control Politics*, 149–50, 153.

65. Midian Othello Bousfield to Michael Marks Davis, Apr. 9, 1932 (quotes 1–2) (MSP-L 31:199); Bousfield, "Negro Public Health Work Needs Birth Control," 170–71 (quotes 3–5).

66. Rodrique, "Afro-American Community," 180–81.

67. Clinics with high percentages of African American patients included North Carolina public health clinics (55 percent), the BCCRB's Harlem Branch (55 percent), Pittsburgh's Irene Kaufmann Settlement House (39 percent), Houston Maternal Health Center (34 percent), Danville, Va., Health Department clinic (32 percent), CMHA clinic (30 percent), and Detroit's North End Clinic (30 percent) and Woman's Hospital Clinic (29 percent). See George M. Cooper, "Birth Control in the North Carolina Health Department," *North Carolina Medical Journal* 1:9 (Sept. 1940): 465; Harlem Branch Statistical Report, Feb. 1, 1930 to Dec. 31, 1930 (MSP-S 61:462); Kaufman Settlement Clinic Annual Report, 1936 (PPWPR); 1935–36 CMHA Annual Report (PPASLR); Pope, "History of Birth Control in Michigan" and "Woman's Hospital Resume of Cases," Apr. 8, 1931 to Aug. 3, 1932 (PPLDR); Rodrique, "Afro-American Community," 152 n. 23; Danville City Health Department Annual Report, 1934 (MSP-L 107:146).

68. Du Bois, "Black Folks and Birth Control," and Johnson, "Question of Negro

Health," as well as Bousfield, "Negro Public Health Work Needs Birth Control," and Fisher, "Negro Social Worker," 175–76.

69. Norman E. Himes, "Clinical Service for the Negro," and Carolyn Bryant, "The Cincinnati Clinic," *BCR* 16:6 (June 1932): 176–77 (quote).

70. The funds came from Clarence Gamble (Leung, "'Better Babies,'" 56–60).

71. Margaret Sanger, Mary Reinhardt Lasker, and Florence Rose, "Birth Control and the Negro," July 1938 (Rose).

72. See Sanger's notation in margin of Florence Rose to Sanger, Nov, 2, 1939 (MSP-S 7:411).

73. PPFA, *Better Health for 13,000,000*, 6.

74. Ibid., 8–10 (quote). For more, see Schoen, *Choice and Coercion*, 49–50, and Norton, "Health Department Birth Control Program."

75. PPFA, *Better Health for 13,000,000*, 11–18.

76. Marie B. Schanks, "Program and Progress on Work with Negroes," Jan. 1945 (PPFAR).

77. See Angela Davis, "Racism, Birth Control, and Reproductive Rights," in *Women, Race, and Class* (New York: Random House, 1981), 213–14; Manning Marable, "Why Black Americans Are Not Socialists," in *Speaking Truth to Power: Essays on Race, Resistance, and Radicalism* (Boulder, Colo.: Westview Press, 1994), 216–17; Angela Franks, *Margaret Sanger's Eugenic Legacy*, 44; and Edwin Black, *War Against the Weak: Eugenics and America's Claim to Create a Master Race* (New York: Thunder's Mouth Press, 2004), 133, 135.

CHAPTER 5: THE CLINIC AND ITS PATIENTS

1. Sanger to Stuart Mudd, July 17, 1929 (MSP-L 28:427–28).

2. Sanger, "Clinics, Courts, and Jails," *BCR* 3:4 (Apr. 1918): 3.

3. There is no basis for questioning the authenticity of these letters. In cases where both the original letter and a published version survive, the editorial changes made were slight (see Margaret Sanger, *Motherhood in Bondage* [New York: Brentano's, 1928], for the largest published collection).

4. For the most important statistical studies, see Kopp, *Birth Control in Practice;* Stix and Notestein, *Controlled Fertility;* Robishaw, "Study of 4,000 Patients," and CMHA, Annual Reports; Planned Parenthood of Pittsburgh, *Changing Clientele.*

5. For Sadie Sachs, see Sanger, *My Fight*, 51–57; Meyer, *Any Friend*, 28–29. Meyer suspects the veracity of this story. See also, "Anti-Birth Control Clinic Is Unmolested," *New York Tribune*, Oct., 24, 1916 (quote), and Bess Scott, "Mother of 11 Children Died and Houston Maternal Health Center Was Born," *Houston Post*, Apr. 3, 1938; also, Anderson, "Private Choices," 1–2.

6. Sanger, *My Fight*, 51–55.

7. Condit, "Underprivileged," 115–17.

8. Anonymous (Mt. Olive, Ark.) to Little Rock Birth Control Clinic, Apr. 1941 (AEAR).

9. Angus McLaren, *History of Contraception: From Antiquity to the Present Day* (Cambridge, Mass.: Blackwell, 1990), 221.

10. The letters published in Sanger's *Motherhood in Bondage*, for example, were grouped in thematic chapters to match topics such as "The Doctor Warns—But Does Not Tell." The largest collection of patient letters can be found in the MSP microfilm, indexed under the name "Client." Other significant gatherings of letters can be found in the AEAR, the Aletta Jacobs Papers (International Informatiecentrum en Archief voor de Vrouwenbewgeing), and the Mary Ware Dennett Papers (Schlesinger Library) reel 18, folders 370–79.

11. Case records of individual patients are extremely rare. Medical records were routinely destroyed and only random samples preserved in archives.

12. Stix and Notestein, *Controlled Fertility*, 167, 120; Robishaw, "Study of 4,000 Patients."

13. The term comes from Christopher Tietze and Robert G. Potter's analysis of various contraceptive methods in the 1950s and 1960s. Seeking to explain and evaluate the high drop-out rate in contraceptive trials, they concluded that women who remained in the trial—the "determined contraceptors"—offered the most accurate gauge of the effectiveness of a contraceptive. Another measure, however, was "use-effectiveness," which calculated in the likelihood that a patient would stick with the method. This allowed differentiation between effective but unpleasant methods. If a method was 100 percent effective, but half the women who tried it discontinued it, its use-effectiveness would be only 50 percent. Long-term clinic patients can be seen as such "determined contraceptors," and their experiences offer a kind of best-case scenario for a method's effectiveness (Meldrum, "'Simple Methods' and 'Determined Contraceptors,'" 289–94).

14. Pearl, "Fertility and Contraception in New York," 1385–90; Robinson, *Seventy Birth Control Clinics*, 65; Stix and Notestein, *Controlled Fertility*, 41–44; Anna E. Nash to MS, May 2, 1929 (quote 1) (MSP-L 32:125); Anonymous (Eaton, Ark.) to Hilda Cornish, Feb. 27, 1940 (quote 2) (AEAR).

15. Sanger, *Motherhood in Bondage*, 40 (quotes 1–2), 45 (quote 3), and 47 (quote 4).

16. Mary Sumner Boyd, "Analysis of Typical Letters," in Sanger, *Motherhood in Bondage*, 443.

17. Chicago's Jewish Social Services Institute Clinic reported 47 percent of its patients had undergone abortions; the Recreation Rooms Settlement Clinic in New York reported 48 percent, and the BCCRB's Harlem Branch reported 42 percent. Other clinics reported smaller figures—only 15 percent for the Los Angeles Mothers' Clinic, for example (Stix and Notestein, *Controlled Fertility*, 12–13; Robinson, *Seventy Birth Control Clinics*, 65; Lamport, "Recreation Rooms"; Los Angeles Mothers' Clinic, "Survey of 3,000 Cases," Apr. 19, 1929 [MSP-L 85:656]).

18. Kopp, *Birth Control in Practice*, 114, appendix 4.

19. In contrast, an analysis of four thousand letters written to Sanger averaged five children in each family, with 12.5 percent having borne over eight children (though new families and those with no children were omitted from the averages). At the Harlem Urban League Center, patients averaged 3.5 pregnancies before attending the clinic, 4.8 in Philadelphia's Maternal Health Center, 4.2 at the South End and Brookline, Massachusetts, clinics. By 1939 the BCFA reported national figures of

2.67 pregnancies for clinic patients (Boyd, "Analysis," 443; Granger, "Birth Control in Harlem," 91–92; Philadelphia Maternal Health Center, Annual Report, 1931 [MSP-L 31:332–35]; Martha G. Waldstein, "A Maternal Health Center Reviews Its Patients," *JOC* 4:11 [Nov. 1939]: 204–9; San Francisco Birth Control Educational Center, Report, 1939 [PPASL]; Planned Parenthood of Pittsburgh, *Changing Clientele;* and Dickinson and Morris, "Birth Control Centers," 591–93).

20. For a take on this phenomenon from the British perspective, see Wally Seccombe, "Starting to Stop: Working-class Fertility Decline in London," *Past and Present* 134 (Feb. 1990): 151–88.

21. Nash, "Planned Parenthood for New York Mothers," 128–29.

22. San Francisco Birth Control Educational Center, Report, 1939 (PPASL); Planned Parenthood of Pittsburgh, *Changing Clientele;* Granger, "Birth Control in Harlem," 91–92; Nash, "Planned Parenthood for New York Mothers," 128–29.

23. Robinson, *Seventy Birth Control Clinics,* 68–69.

24. Stix and Notestein, *Controlled Fertility,* 107–10.

25. Bocker, "Birth Control Methods," Kopp, *Birth Control in Practice,* 133; Stix and Notestein, *Controlled Fertility,* 23.

26. Bocker, "Birth Control Methods," 2–8.

27. Kopp, *Birth Control in Practice,* 134.

28. Meldrum, "'Simple Methods' and 'Determined Contraceptors.'"

29. Kopp, *Birth Control in Practice,* 137–39; for a description of problems with an intrauterine "wishbone" pessary, see Sanger, *Motherhood in Bondage,* 311.

30. Robishaw, "Study of 4,000 Patients," 8–10; Stix and Notestein, *Controlled Fertility,* 107–10.

31. Anonymous (Gassville, Ark.) to Arkansas State Hygenics Department, May 7, 1939 (AEAR).

32. Tone, *Devices and Desires,* 151–82.

33. Robinson, *Seventy Birth Control Clinics,* 89, 97–98.

34. Stix and Notestein, *Controlled Fertility,* 12; Leung, "'Better Babies,'" 144, 168–69; Philadelphia Maternal Health Center, 1931 Annual Report (MSP-L 31:332–35); Lamport, "Recreation Rooms"; Minnesota Birth Control League, 1932–33 Annual Report; Monroe County Birth Control League, Annual Report, 1937; and Pittsburgh Maternal Health Clinic, Annual Report, 1936 (PPASLR).

35. "Clinic Reports: Birth Control Educational Center," *JOC* 3:3 (Mar. 1938): 68–71.

36. Anne Kennedy found that almost 93 percent of Chicago patients were housewives; those that worked did so only because they had to. The BCCRB reported 86 percent of its patients were housewives. In Pittsburgh it was 97 percent. By contrast, about 25 percent of women who wrote Sanger for birth control information worked for wages (Kopp, *Birth Control in Practice,* 5–8, and appendix table 4; Anne Kennedy, "A Visit to the Medical Centers of Chicago," *BCR* 10:1 [Jan. 1927]: 26; Meyer, "Birth Control Policy," 171; Planned Parenthood of Pittsburgh, *Changing Clientele;* Boyd, "Analysis," 442; Robinson, *Seventy Birth Control Clinics,* 94).

37. Boyd, "Analysis," 440–42.

38. Dickinson and Morris, "Birth Control Centers," 591–93.

39. Robinson, *Seventy Birth Control Clinics*, 89–94; Holz, "Birth Control Clinic in America," 45.

40. Sanger, "Prolific Child-Breeding Scored by Mrs. Sanger," *San Francisco Call and Post*, June 10, 1916.

41. Leung, "'Better Babies,'" 146. It is difficult to compare these kinds of figures across clinics, for many clinics and states restricted admission to women with medical indications only.

42. Sanger, *Motherhood in Bondage*, 39.

43. "A Day with Margaret Sanger in her Birth Control Clinic," *Brooklyn Daily Eagle*, Oct. 24, 1916.

44. Sanger, *Motherhood in Bondage*, 70–71.

45. Kopp, *Birth Control in Practice*, 41. For examples of letters written to Sanger describing such cases, see chapter 15, "The Doctor Warns—But Does Not Tell," in Sanger, *Motherhood in Bondage*, 359–93.

46. Kopp, *Birth Control in Practice*, 42.

47. Sanger, *Motherhood in Bondage*, 127.

48. Ibid., 288.

49. See Katharine Bement Davis, *Factors in the Sex Lives of Twenty-Two Hundred Women* (New York: Harper and Row, 1929); Cynthia Eagle Russert, *Sexual Science: The Victorian Construction of Womanhood* (Cambridge: Harvard University Press, 1989); Gordon, *Moral Property*, 62–64, 122–35; John d'Emilio and Estelle B. Freedman, *Intimate Matters: A History of Sexuality in America* (Chicago: University of Chicago Press, 1997); Kathy Peiss, *Cheap Amusements: Working Women and Leisure in Turn of the Century New York* (Philadelphia: Temple University Press, 1986). Elizabeth Alice Clement, in *Love for Sale: Courting, Treating, and Prostitution in New York City, 1900–1945* (Chapel Hill: University of North Carolina Press, 2007), concludes that while many single women took part in sexual activities before marriage, many would stop short of intercourse (66–67).

50. Peiss's *Cheap Amusements* covered the working-class culture of unmarried girls from 1880 to 1920. Other studies of immigrants in this period also depict a generational divide between Americanized daughters and more traditional parents. In *Love for Sale*, Clement analyzes changing dating practices, but does not examine sex within working-class marriages.

51. Anonymous (Easton, Ark.) to Hilda Cornish, Feb. 27, 1940 (AEAR).

52. Sanger, *Happiness in Marriage*, 140.

53. See Raymond Pearl, *The Biology of Population Growth* (New York: Alfred A. Knopf, 1925), 186–89.

54. Sanger, *Motherhood in Bondage*, 269.

55. Kopp, *Birth Control in Practice*, 101–3.

56. Anonymous (Logansport, Ind.) to Sanger, Aug. 14, 1924 (MSP-S 2:623).

57. Sanger, *Family Limitation*, 6–7.

58. Gordon, *Moral Property*, 62–64.

59. No resolution of this case survives.

60. The primary fault in men was that they wanted sex more often than their wives did. The Stones reported that a sex frequency from two to three times per week was typical, but recommended that couples follow their "natural desire and capacity to control the frequency of relations." They argued that men were usually the initiators in sexual matters, while women were more passive, a condition reinforced through cultural mores. Women's sexuality was described as "often latent or dormant," only to be awakened over time (Abraham and Hannah M. Stone, *Marriage Manual*, 253–55, 287–88).

61. Marcus eventually sought out additional training in psychology and sex in order to better answer these questions (Chesler, "Sarah Marcus Interview," 26–27.)

62. Marjorie Prevost, "Consultations," Feb. 15, 1932 (MSP-U).

63. Ibid., Feb. 24, 1932 (MSP-U).

64. Ibid., Mar. 20, 1932 (MSP-U).

65. Kopp, *Birth Control in Practice*, 101–3.

66. Sanger, *Motherhood in Bondage*, 337, 354 (quote).

67. Ibid., 339.

68. Ibid., 265 (quote); see also, Sanger, *Happiness in Marriage*, 136–49.

69. Sanger, *Motherhood in Bondage*, 303.

70. Ibid., 272, 281 (quote).

71. See for instance, Schoen, *Choice and Coercion*, 55; Prevost, "Consultations," Feb. 17, 1932 (MSP-U).

72. Effie Lyon to Margaret M. Coghlan, Apr. 25, 1934 (PPASLR).

73. See the Chicago Woman's Aid Society Annual Reports for IBCL Medical Center Five, Apr. 15, 1936 and Apr. 16, 1936 (quote 1) (CWASR); Ann Warner to Helen S. Buss, Oct. 27, 1939 (quote 2) (PPASLR).

74. Marion Warren to Sanger, Nov. 28, 1931 (quotes), and Sanger to Warren, Jan. 13, 1932 (MSP-L 32:455–56).

75. Anna E. Nash to Margaret Sanger, May 2 and May 14, 1929, and Sanger to Nash, May 8 and May 13, 1929 (MSP-L 32:125–28).

76. Florence Revelle to Sanger, Sept. 28, 1931 (MSP-L 29:373).

77. Sanger to Hannah Stone, Sept. 30, 1931 (quote 2), and Sanger to Revelle, Sept. 29 (quote 1) and Oct. 29, 1931 (quote 3) (MSP-L 29:385–88).

78. Pasadena Hospital Clinic, "Increasing Clinic Attendance," 1–2.

79. Most clinics recorded the religions of their patients. Despite the opposition of the Catholic Church, Catholic women attended clinics as easily as those of other religions. It was not until the late 1940s that the PPFA stopped asking patients their religions (Sanger to Abraham Stone, n.d. [MSP-C 11:798]; Kopp, *Birth Control in Practice*, 51–52; Robinson, *Seventy Birth Control Clinics*, 62; Planned Parenthood of Pittsburgh, *Changing Clientele;* IBCL, Annual Reports, 1930–38; Leung, "'Better Babies,'" 169; and ABCL, Annual Report, 1937, 29 [PPFAR]).

80. Sanger to Abraham Stone, ca. 1940 (MSP-C C11:798).

81. Prevost to Sanger, May 4, 1932 (MSP-L 32:264–65).

82. Rodrique, "Afro-American Community," 153.

83. Ruth Topping, "Memo to Files," Mar. 27, 1931 (BSHR); McCann, *Birth Control Politics*, 80–81.

84. Lenore Guttmacher, "Securing Patients for a Rural Center," *BCR* 22:11 (Nov. 1938): 130–31.

85. Marguerite Martin, "In Behalf of Mothers," *St. Louis Post-Dispatch*, Mar. 31, 1937; Tasker, "Mothers' Clinic," 251–52; Sanger to Lawrence Dunham, July 31, 1928 (MSP-L 35:161); Planned Parenthood Clinic of Pittsburgh, *Changing Clientele.*

86. Tasker, "Mothers' Clinic," 251–52; "A Statistical Evaluation of the Follow-Up Work of the Maternal Health Association of Missouri for the Year 1938" (quote) (PPASLR).

87. Kopp, *Birth Control in Practice*, 37; Dickinson and Morris, "Birth Control Centers," 591–93.

88. Elizabeth Watson, "Spreading the News," *BCR* 9:6 (June 1926): 192.

89. Etta Hediger, Report on the Brooklyn Branch of the BCCRB, in "News Notes," *BCR* 9:10 (Oct. 1926): 318; Hart, "Homes of the Poor," 319–20.

90. "Mrs. Sanger's Aid Found Guilty," *New York Times*, Jan. 9, 1917 (quote 1); "Senators Hear Mother Tell How Birth Data Saved Her," *Chicago Daily Tribune*, Mar. 2, 1934 (quote 2).

91. Pringle, "Women of America," 14; "Clinical Contraception in the United States," *JOC* 4:8 (Aug.–Sept. 1939): 168–69.

CHAPTER 6: CLINICS AND THE FEDERAL GOVERNMENT

1. "Sanger Calls on U.S.," *New York Herald Tribune*, Oct. 6, 1938.

2. The Comstock Law banned: "Every obscene, lewd, or lascivious, and every filthy, book, pamphlet, picture, paper, letter, writing, print, or other publication of an indecent character, and every article or thing designed, adapted, or intended for preventing conception or producing abortion, or for any indecent or immoral use; and every article, instrument, substance, drug, medicine, or thing which is advertised or described in a manner calculated to lead another to use or apply it for preventing conception or producing abortion, or for any indecent or immoral purpose" (U.S. Criminal Code, Section 211 [1909]; Janet Brodie, *Contraception and Abortion*, Beisel, *Imperiled Innocents*, and Garrow, *Liberty and Sexuality;* for its implementation in the twentieth century, see Dienes, *Law, Politics, and Birth Control*, and Dennett, *Birth Control Laws.*

3. For the complete texts of federal and state laws, see BCCRB, *Laws Relating to Birth Control in the U.S. and Its Territories* (New York: BCCRB, 1938), 10–16.

4. *Family Limitation* was the most obvious of these materials, and Sanger revised and reprinted it throughout the 1930s. Three other pamphlets, *English Methods of Birth Control*, *Dutch Methods of Birth Control*, and *Magnetation Methods of Birth Control* (all 1915), also included practical advice. Sanger also published lists of birth control clinics in the *BCR*. In 1926, her husband's lawyer, Newell W. Ellison, advised her

that such mailings clearly violated the Comstock Act, but she ignored his warnings (Newell W. Ellison to J. Noah Slee and Sanger, Oct. 18, 1926 [MSP-L 11:664]).

5. Dennett, *Birth Control Laws*, and Chen, *Sex Side of Life*. For Dennett's congressional diaries, see Dennett microfilm, reels 12–13, folders 240–48.

6. For an overview of the NCFLBC's work, see NCFLBC, *New Day Dawns;* for the reactions of congressmen, see the NCFLBC's congressional reports (MSP-L reels 77–83).

7. McCann, *Birth Control Politics*, 63–64.

8. Alvah Sulloway, "The Legal and Political Aspects of Population Control in the United States," *Law and Contemporary Problems* 25:3 (Summer 1960): 602 (quote); Dienes, *Law, Politics, and Birth Control*, 113–14; Chesler, *Woman of Valor*, 373–76.

9. Paul S. Boyer, *Purity in Print: The Vice-Society Movement and Book Censorship in America* (New York: Scribner, 1968), 74, 99, 129, 248, 253; Robert A. Liston, *The Right to Know: Censorship in America* (New York: F. Watts, 1973), 24–28; Morris L. Ernst and Alan U. Schwartz, *Censorship: The Search for the Obscene* (New York: Macmillan, 1964), 62. See also "Publishers Oppose Clean Books Bill," and "Clean Books Bill Dies in the Senate," *New York Times*, Apr. 24 and May 3, 1923.

10. Newell W. Ellison to J. Noah Slee and Sanger, Oct. 18, 1926 (MSP-L 11:664); Chesler, *Woman of Valor*, 317.

11. Tresca was arrested in 1923 for publishing an advertisement for a contraceptive book in *Il Martello*, his anarchist journal ("Coolidge Reduces the Sentence of Tresca," *New York Times*, Feb. 17, 1925).

12. Most manufacturers got around the law by describing their products as feminine hygiene aids. Sanger had difficulty importing and exporting the proceedings of contraceptive conferences, samples of contraceptives, and books on birth control (Tone, *Devices and Desires*, 151–82; see NCFLBC Legal Files, MSP-L reels 58–60).

13. The NCFLBC's bill was designed as the first in a number of incremental steps that would eventually legalize contraception. Pragmatic, Sanger believed that there was no political support for a complete repeal of the Comstock Act, and that the more limited doctors-only bill, with the backing of the medical profession, women's groups, and social workers had a chance to pass (Chen, *Sex Side of Life*, 223–38; see Katz, *Selected Papers*, vols. 1 and 2).

14. After the 1934 defeat of S.1842, the NCFLBC began putting more emphasis on grassroots campaigning, securing endorsements, and creating petitions to pressure the White House, rather than debating congressmen directly (see Hazel Moore, "Lobbying Report," June 13, 1934, Sanger to Moore, Sept. 4, 1935 and Oct. 11, 1935, and Moore to Sanger, Sept. 28, 1935 [MSP-L 68:349B, MSP-S 10:338, 448, and 390]; Katz, *Selected Papers*, vol. 2.)

15. Judge Grover Moscowitz dismissed the case on January 6, 1936. The U.S. appealed and the Second Circuit Court of Appeals decided the case on December 7, 1936 (Greenbaum, Wolff, and Ernst, "Summary of Brief for Claimant-Appellate," Oct. 5, 1936 [MSP-L 60:262]; Dienes, *Law, Politics, and Birth Control*, 112, quoting Judge Augustus Hand's majority opinion).

16. Birth Control Council of America, minutes, May 5, May 14, June 1 and 27, 1937 (PPLMR; MSP-S 62:13, MSP-L 32:209A, MSP-S 62:6).

17. Dienes, *Law, Politics, and Birth Control,* 116.

18. Amy Sarch, "Dirty Discourse: Birth Control Advertising in the 1920s and 1930s," Ph.D. diss., University of Pennsylvania, 1994; Robyn Rosen, "Federal Expansion, Fertility Control, and Physicians in the United States: The Politics of Motherhood in the Interwar Years," *Journal of Women's History* 10:3 (Autumn 1983): 53–73; Pringle, "Women of America," 14–15, 94.

19. Dorothy Kenyon, "Nullification or Repeal," *BCR* 14:10 (Oct. 1930): 278–80; Eleanor Dwight Jones, "The American Birth Control Movement," *BCR* 15:12 (Dec. 1931): 341–42.

20. See Sanger to Agnes Smedley, Jan. 8, 1925, and J. Noah Slee to Hechtel Ie Noir and Murray Agency, Oct. 16, 1924 and Nov. 10, 1924 (MSP-L 10:293 and 11:579, 582).

21. Lenore Schwab Black (1874–1955) was vice chairman of the CMHA and a member of its board of trustees (Nancy Peacock, "Everything you Wanted to Know about Noblesse Oblige But Were Afraid to Ask," *Cleveland* (May 1998): 96; Meyer, *Any Friend,* 70).

22. Contraceptive manufacturers used euphemisms and the catchall term "feminine hygiene" to avoid prosecution under the Comstock Act. All that was needed was an alternate use for the contraceptive, such as the use of a condom to avert venereal disease or the use of a diaphragm as a "womb supporter," to use the mails for "legitimate" purposes (Tone, *Devices and Desires,* 152–53).

23. Harry M. Fisher, "Birth Control and Public Policy," *BCR* 5:7 (June 1924): 165–68. In Sacramento, the district attorney threatened to prosecute the clinic if it violated the law by making any public announcements. This effort to dissuade the activists from opening succeeded from 1937 to 1940 (Cele Damon to Bernice Wickham, June 14, 1937, Gladys DeLancey Smith, "Special Interview," July 10, 1938, and report on Irene Mugford, Apr. 20, 1938 [MSP-L 33:707B, 39:381, 377]).

24. Cora Meyer to theACLU, Mar. 25, 1935 (ACLUR); Holz, "Nurse Gordon on Trial," 112–40.

25. "Police in Boston Raid Birth League," *New York Times,* Aug. 4, 1937.

26. The clinics that closed were: the Brownsville Clinic (1916), the Brookline, Salem, Fitchburg, Springfield, Worcester, and New Bedford Mothers' Health Offices of the Massachusetts Birth Control League (1937), and the New Haven, Hartford, Greenwich, Norwalk, Danbury, Westport, Stanford, and New Britain branches of the Connecticut Maternal Health League (1940). Nurse Adele Gordon's Milwaukee Medical Bureau of Information closed shortly after her acquittal, for unknown reasons (George A. Bowman to Samuel Paul Puner, Apr. 5, 1935 [ACLUR]; for extensive correspondence on the Gordon case, see MSP-L 108:210–89; Holz, "Nurse Gordon on Trial," 112).

27. The BCCRB raid took place on April 15, 1929, at the instigation of local Catholic officials. Doctors Hannah Stone and Elizabeth Pissoort were arrested, along with nurses Sigrid Brestwell, Marcella Sideri, and Antoinette Field. The police also confiscated medical supplies, six patient records, and patient information cards. All charges were dismissed on May 14, as Magistrate Abraham Rosenbluth ruled that

the BCCRB acted in good faith in prescribing contraceptives to a married woman for health reasons ("Raid Sanger Clinic on Birth Control," *New York Times*, Apr. 16, 1929; Sanger, *Autobiography*, 404–5; "Judge Rosenbluth's Opinion," *BCR* 12:7 [July 1929]: 194).

28. Sanger served thirty days without incident, but Byrne was released early due to her deteriorating condition following a highly publicized hunger strike (Sanger, "Clinics, Courts, and Jails").

29. Stone, "Massachusetts Raid," 181.

30. Dienes, *Law, Politics, and Birth Control*, 117, 137.

31. In Massachusetts, medical and lay staff were arrested, tried, and convicted. On appeal, the BCLM argued that physicians should be exempt, but the State Supreme Court denied their appeal, indicating that the law made no exceptions for physicians. Any change in the wording of the law had to come from legislative reform. After the trial, the BCLM attempted, without success, to overturn the law. For an overview of the Massachusetts raids and closing, see ABCL, Annual Report, 1937, 31 (PPFAR), and "Birth Control and the Massachusetts Law" (PPLMR); Stone, "Massachusetts Raid," 181 (quote); "Waterbury Clinic Report," June 27, 1939 (PPFAR), and "Worksheet for Clinic History" (PPWPR); Garrow, *Liberty and Sexuality*, 2–8, 63.

32. "'Totalitarians' Called U.S. Foes of Birth Control," *New York Herald Tribune*, Sept. 6, 1941 (quote); George Gallup, "The Gallup Poll: Birth Control Information through Public Health Clinics Favored in Survey," *Washington Post*, Jan. 24, 1940.

33. After the *One Package* decision, Sanger reported that birth control dissemination was legal in twenty-one states. In ten, physicians were exempt from obscenity laws, and contraceptives could be sold in drug stores. In three, physicians were exempt, but druggists were not. In six, contraceptives could not be "indiscriminately" advertised or distributed (Sanger, "Status of Birth Control: 1938," *New Republic*, Apr. 20, 1938 [MSP-C 16:417]).

34. In Cleveland, women became active in 1921, when Dorothy Brush attended Sanger's First American Birth Control Conference in New York City. They investigated the laws and decided that physicians could give advice as long as they did not use the mails. Brush and others formed the CMHA in 1923 and then tried to convince a hospital to offer birth control services. Failing that, they finally opened their own clinic in 1928. Similarly, the Detroit Birth Control League, formed in 1922, did not open its first clinic for five years (Meyer, *Any Friend*, 28–29, 33, 44–48; Guttmacher, *Planned Parenthood Beginnings*, 103, 58.)

35. Sanger's Brownsville clinic appeal broadened New York State law in 1918 when Judge Crane exempted physicians who prescribed contraceptives for the cure and prevention of disease. Sanger sought to broaden the ruling in 1919 and 1922, by extending protection to nurses and legalizing contraception for economic and social reasons. By 1923, she backed down on the former, but continued to press to allow doctors to prescribe birth control for any reason they saw fit. This remained her legislative policy throughout the 1920s and 1930s, forming the basis of her state and federal lobbying and of the clinic standards she exported to leagues in the United States and abroad (Katz, *Selected Papers* 1:394).

36. After 1923, Sanger argued that contraceptives should only be prescribed by physicians. As late as 1950, she wrote to Abraham Stone about the Tucson clinic: "The nurse here we discovered has been fitting diaphragms for two years—sometimes it is too small & then she calls the Doctor but one of the Doctors a woman with Mexican practice winked her eye at this & said 'I told the nurse to go ahead & finish up.' . . . I want a medical decision on this Abraham from your medical group or the PPF group—we either uphold the standards we set years ago or turn the whole thing over to unprofessionals. Let me have your opinion and action." No response was found (Sanger to Stone, ca. 1950 [MSP-C 11:807]).

37. The American government was far slower to address issues of infant and maternal mortality than other industrialized nations. It did not offer public health programs or other poverty reducing programs until the 1920s (Meckel, *Save the Babies*, 134; U.S. Census Bureau, *Historical Statistics of the U.S.* [Washington: GPO, 1975], 57).

38. Lara Marks, *Metropolitan Maternity: Maternal and Infant Mortality in Early 20th Century London* (Atlanta: Rodopi, 1996), 89, 114; Loudon, "Deaths in Childbed from the 18th Century to 1935," *Medical History* 30:1 [Jan. 1986]: 1–41).

39. Meckel, *Save the Babies*, 160–79; Irvine Loudon, "Some international features of maternal mortality, 1880–1950," in Valerie Fildes, Lara Marks, and Hilary Marland, eds., *Women and Children First: International Maternal and Infant Welfare, 1870–1945* (New York: Routledge, 1992), 17–21.

40. Robert Woodbury, *Causal Factors in Infant Mortality* (Washington: GPO, 1925), 48, 60–61; U.S. Children's Bureau, *Conference on Better Care for Mothers and Babies* (Washington: GPO, 1938), 7, 38; Sanger, "Status of Birth Control: 1938"; Meckel, *Save the Babies*, 153; Mary Alden Hopkins, "Dead Babies," *Harpers Weekly*, Apr. 17, 1915, 370; Robinson, *Seventy Birth Control Clinics*, 65; "Editorials: Contraception among Urban Populations," *JOC* 2:5 (May 1937): 110–11.

41. For histories of the PHS and CB, see Mullan, *Plagues and Politics;* Robyn Muncy, *Creating a Female Dominion in American Reform, 1890–1935* (New York: Oxford University Press, 1991), 51–56; James Leiby, *A History of Social Welfare and Social Work in the United States* (New York: Columbia University Press, 1978), 286.

42. See Elizabeth Fee, "Public Health and the State: The United States," in Porter, ed., *The History of Public Health and the Modern State*, 229–31, 243–45; Meckel, *Save the Babies*, 126–28.

43. Paul V. Starr, *Social Transformation of American Medicine* (New York: Basic Books, 1982), 252–66, 270–75.

44. The CB worked with local women's groups to gather detailed data, which was then published in a series of case studies on *Infant Mortality*. Reports came from Johnstown, Pa. (1915), Manchester, N.H. (1917), Waterbury, Conn. (1918), Saginaw, Mich. (1919), Akron, Ohio (1920), Pittsburgh, Pa. (1921), Gary, Ind. (1923), Baltimore, Md. (1923), Memphis, Tenn. (1937), and others.

45. Ladd-Taylor, *Raising a Baby*, 13–23.

46. Meckel, *Save the Babies*, 131–32; Ladd-Taylor, *Raising a Baby*, 25–27; Rothman, *Woman's Proper Place*, 136–38.

47. McCann, *Birth Control Politics*, 52–53.

48. Massachusetts, Connecticut, and Illinois declined to pass legislation needed to receive federal funding (Ladd-Taylor, *Raising a Baby*, 28).

49. In North Carolina, the state used Sheppard-Towner funding to create a Bureau of Maternity and Infancy, which employed doctors and nurses to instruct impoverished women on prenatal and infant hygiene, conduct midwife training, and visit pregnant women and those who had recently had babies (Schoen, *Choice and Coercion*, 27).

50. Rosen, "Federal Expansion, Fertility Control, and Physicians in the United States: The Politics of Motherhood in the Interwar Years," *Journal of Women's History* 10:3 (Autumn 1998): 61–63.

51. Rothman, *Woman's Proper Place*, 142–46.

52. Ladd-Taylor, *Raising a Baby*, 30–31; Schoen, *Choice and Coercion*, 27.

53. Quoted in Mullan, *Plagues and Politics*, 59.

54. Chesler, *Woman of Valor*, 378.

55. For more on this see Mullan, *Plagues and Politics*, 109–10.

56. For efforts to include birth control in Georgia's public health program, see E. Bouton to Mrs. Conrad, June 25, 1939, and "Summary of B.C. in Public Health," presented at the Institute, Sept. 1939 (PPFAR); for South Carolina, see "South Carolina Adds Birth Control to its Public Health Program," *BCR* 4:12 (Dec. 1939): 27, and BCFA, "Parenthood U.S.A.—The Story of South Carolina," 1942 (MSP-C 14:91); for Farm Security Administration efforts among migrant workers in California, see Gordon, *Moral Property*, 237.

57. Fee, "Public Health and the State," 246–47.

58. See Chesler, *Woman of Valor*, 377. In the 1940s, the CB agreed to release Social Security funds for contraceptive services, though few requests were made for them. In 1941, Lenroot "expressed fear that inclusion of birth control would jeopardize her other programs of maternal and child welfare" ("Margaret Sanger Calls on the U.S. to Offer Birth Control Service," *New York Herald Tribune*, Oct. 6, 1938; see MS to Committee on Public Progress member, Feb. 11, 1938, and Reference Sheet on Public Progress letters to Thomas Parran, ca. 1938, and Katharine Lenroot to Lawrence T. Smith, Mar. 3, 1938 [MSP-S 61:878, MSP-L 115:319, 115A]; Reed, *Birth Control Movement*, 267–68).

59. ABCL Annual Report, 1937; Eric Matsner, "Annual Report of the ABCL Medical Department," 1937 (PPFAR).

60. ABCL, "Suggested Methods of Conducting Contraceptive Instruction Under Health Department Auspices," Mar. 1938 (PPFAR).

61. See McCann, *Birth Control Politics*, 199–200; ABCL Annual Report, 1938, 7–8 (PPFAR); "The Children's Bureau Conference," *BCR* 22:2 (Feb. 1938): 47–48; and Sanger to Mary Winsor, May 3, 1939 (quote) (MSP-S 16:783).

CHAPTER 7: LOCAL CLINICS AND NATIONAL ORGANIZATIONS

1. See Gordon, *Moral Property*, Reed, *Birth Control Movement*, and McCann, *Birth Control Politics*.

2. See, among others, Caron, *Who Chooses?*, Meyer, *Any Friend*, and Leung, "'Better Babies.'"

3. Special Meeting of the ABCL Board of Directors, Oct. 31, 1935 (MSP-L 28:38), and BCFA Citizen's Committee for Planned Parenthood, 1940 (MSP-S 62:67).

4. NCFLBC, *New Day Dawns*, 25.

5. Ibid.; BCFA, "Objectives," Feb. 1939 (MSP-S 62:36); Elizabeth Beeson, "Meetings of the Executive Secretaries of State Birth Control Leagues," May 30, 1940 (PPFAR); and ABCL Annual Reports (PPFAR).

6. For examples, see Gordon, *Moral Property*, 187–88, 205, and Reed, *Birth Control Movement*, 107–28.

7. By 1935, the BCCRB and NCFLBC Executive Committees met in joint sessions, while in the 1920s, the BCCRB was so entangled with the ABCL that Sanger faced difficulties when she left in 1928 in taking the clinic with her (NCFLBC/BCCRB Minutes, Dec. 6, 1935, and Jan. 3, 1936 [MSP-S 64:548, 553]; Sanger to Juliet Rublee, Sept. 23, 1928 [MSP-C 4:740]).

8. See Guttmacher, *Planned Parenthood Beginnings*, and the state appendices to Vreeland, "Process of Reform," for histories of many state and local leagues and clinics.

9. "Some History of Birth Control in Chicago," n.d. (quote 1) (MS Unfilmed); "Margaret H. Cohn Dies, Cultural, Rights Leader," *Buffalo News*, Oct. 7, 1994 (quote 2).

10. Meyer, *Any Friend*, 32–35; Robinson, *Seventy Birth Control Clinics*, 30; "Middlebury People Start First Vermont Birth Control Council," *Middlebury Register*, Aug. 9, 1935 (Upson).

11. James Freyer Cooper's reports from Jan. 1925 to Dec. 1926 are filmed on MSP-C 12:56–447. For ABCL field work, see MSP-L reel 27; NCFLBC field work reports are filmed by state on MSP-L reels 83–108; see ABCL, 1937 Annual Report (PPFAR).

12. For examples, see Vreeland, "Process of Reform," Michigan appendix, and Katz, *Selected Papers* 1:262–66.

13. The best coverage of Sanger's speaking appearances from 1917 through 1928 can be found in the *BCR* column, "News Notes," which provides details on the audiences and themes of her appearances. The texts of her extant speeches are filmed in MSP-L, reels 128–31, MSP-S reels 70–77, and MSP-C, reel 16.

14. Robinson, "How Shall We Start a Clinic?" 143–44.

15. Pope, "Story of Birth Control in Michigan, 1922 to 1943" (PPLDR) (quote); Guttmacher, *Planned Parenthood Beginnings*, 58; Vreeland, "Process of Reform," Michigan appendix.

16. Sanger to Marjorie Prevost, Jan. 27, 1932 (MSP-L 32:213).

17. Ibid. (quote 1); Kate Belcher, "High Lights in High Spots," ca. Sept. 1927 (other quotes) (PPFAR), and Guttmacher, *Planned Parenthood Beginnings*, 67–70.

18. For a sample of lecture requests, see correspondence with the Margaret Sanger Lecture Bureau, ca. 1921, and the ABCL (ABCLR), and for requests from 1936 through 1954, see MSP-L reels 58, and 131–34.

19. Robinson, "How Shall We Start a Clinic?" 143–44; BCCRB, "How to Establish a Birth Control Clinic"; Sanger to Prevost, Jan. 27, 1932 (quote) (MSP-L 32:213).

20. Indianapolis Maternal Health League minutes, June 4 and Nov. 26, 1934, and Feb. 25 and Mar. 25, 1935 (quote) (PPCIR).

21. These directories are the best source of detail on when clinics were in operation and when they closed.

22. Sanger to Mrs. Dan Jones, Sept. 7, 1935 (MSP-L 7:614); Richard Pierson to Cele Damon, Feb. 8, 1938 (PPFAR).

23. ABCL Board of Directors Meeting, Mar. 2, 1933 (PPLMR); McCann, *Birth Control Politics*, 181–83; IBCL Annual Report, 1937 (PPASLR). See also the work on Ruth Smith in Nebraska and Indiana, in Reports of Nebraska Maternal Health Association and Maternal Health League of Indiana to the ABCL, 1936 (PPFAR).

24. Hannah Stone, "A Clinic Questionnaire," *BCR* 17:4 (Apr. 1934): 3; Sanger to Elizabeth Bacon, Sept. 5, 1935 (MSP-L 95:125); Sanger, "Clinic Affiliation," Sept. 2, 1935 (MSP-S 60:275).

25. NCFLBC, *New Day Dawns*, 58; NCLFBC, "Birth Control Newsletter," June 1935, and "Third Newsletter," June 9, 1930 (MSP-S 64:811 and 790).

26. ABCL, "Why Affiliate?"; Marguerite Benson to Clarence Gamble, Oct. 8, 1935 (PPFAR).

27. ABCL, "Why Affiliate?"

28. McCann, *Birth Control Politics*, 181–84; Gordon, *Moral Property*, 205–10; and ABCL Board of Directors Minutes, May 23, 1935 (MSP-L 28:33).

29. Eric Matsner, ABCL Medical Director's Report, Sept. 15 through Nov. 25, 1936 (PPFAR).

30. ABCL Annual Report, 1938 (PPFAR).

31. Sanger to Hannah Stone, Jan. 31, 1933 (MSP-L 32:381–82).

32. Dickinson to Sanger, Sept. 16, 1941 (MSP-S 19:941), Knopf to Sanger, Feb. 21, 1929 (quote 1), and Sanger to Elizabeth Bacon, Sept. 5, 1935 (quote 2) (MSP-L 57:344 and 95:125).

33. "News Items," *JOC* 2:11 (Nov. 1936): 199.

34. The foam powder testing was carried out both in the United States and abroad, in an effort to find an effective contraceptive that did not require fitting by a physician (Cele Damon to Charlotte Noland, Nov. 16, 1936 [MSP-L 107:114]).

35. "News Notes: Clinic Exchange," *JOC* 3:2 (Feb. 1937): 48.

36. BCCRB, "How to Establish a Birth Control Clinic."

37. Ibid.

38. Sanger, "Open Letter"; "Standards for Affiliated Clinics," n.d. (MSP-U).

39. Sanger to Mary Hughston, Sept. 5, 1935 (MSP-L 83:620).

40. Eric Matsner to Maurice Newfield, May 21, 1937 (PPFAR).

41. ABCL Annual Report, 1937 (PPFAR).

42. Sanger to Hilda Cornish, Apr. 24, 1933 (MSP-L 84:451).

43. Eric Matsner to Maurice Newfield, May 21, 1937 (PPFAR).

44. Indianapolis Maternal Heath League, Board of Directors minutes, Nov. 27, 1933, Dec. 4, 1933, Apr. 2, 1934, and Oct. 8, 1934 (quote) (PPCIR).

45. Donald West to Clarence Gamble, Sept. 5, 1933 (Gamble); Meyer, *Any Friend*, 74; Norman Himes and Abraham Stone, *Practical Birth-Control Methods* (New York: Viking, 1942), 205.

46. The CMHA's members may have held a grudge against the ABCL for its treatment of Sanger, but they did not affiliate with the BCCRB either. They also resisted aligning themselves with medical organizations, out of fear that it would divide the association along religious lines (Meyer, "Birth Control Policy," 89–90).

47. Sanger to D. Kenneth Rose, Nov. 5, 1939 (MSP-S 17:420).

48. Sanger to Hilda Cornish, Dec. 30, 1933 (MSP-L 84:466); Richard Pierson to Cele Damon, Feb. 8, 1938 (PPFAR).

49. In 1937 the total was up to 207, but with the two-year certificates the ABCL only secured 107 affiliated clinics in 1938 (Alison Moore, "Report for 1936," read at ABCL Annual Meeting, Jan. 28, 1937; ABCL Annual Reports, 1937 and 1938 [PPFAR]).

50. Sanger, "Clinic Affiliations," Sept. 25, 1935 (MSP-S 61:275), and Hazel Zborowski to Sanger, May 1, 1936 (MSP-L 34:642).

51. Sanger, "Open Letter."

52. For examples, see Garrow, *Liberty and Sexuality*, 80–83, and Sanger to Rosalyn Weir, Mar. 2, 1950 (MSP-L 119:218).

CONCLUSION

1. Sanger to Juliet Rublee, Aug. 10, 1918 (MSP-C 1:281).

2. This was the title of a 1911 series of columns, published in the *New York Call* and as a stand-alone pamphlet, imparting sex education lectures for mothers to impart to their children. It was followed by the series "What Every Girl Should Know," which launched Sanger into the fight against censorship in 1913.

Bibliography

Published sources cited more than once appear in shortened format in the notes and are expanded here; sources that appear only one time are fully cited in the notes section for each chapter.

ARCHIVAL COLLECTIONS

American Civil Liberties Papers (ACLUR), Princeton University, Sealey G. Mudd Library.

Arkansas Eugenics Association Records (AEAR), University of Arkansas for Medical Sciences Library.

Bureau of Social Hygiene Records (BSHR), Rockefeller Archive Center.

Chicago Woman's Aid Records (CWASR), University of Illinois, Chicago.

Papers of Mary Ware Dennett and the Voluntary Parenthood League (Dennett Microfilm), Part B of Women's studies manuscript collections from the Schlesinger Library, Radcliffe College. Series 3: Sexuality, Sex education, and Reproductive Rights (Bethesda, Md.: University Publications of America, 1994).

Clarence Gamble Papers (Gamble), Countway Library of Medicine.

Adolf Meyer Papers (Meyer), Alan Mason McChesney Medical Archives, Johns Hopkins University.

National Committee on Maternal Health Records (NCMHR), Countway Library of Medicine.

Frances Noel Papers (Noel), UCLA Special Collections.

J. W. R. Norton Papers (Norton), University of North Carolina–Chapel Hill, Southern Historical Collection.

Office of the Messrs. Rockefeller, Medical Interests Series (OMRR), Rockefeller Archive Center.

Florence Rose Papers (Rose), Sophia Smith Collection, Smith College.

Planned Parenthood Association of Central Indiana Records (PPCIR), Indiana Historical Society Library.

Planned Parenthood Association of St. Louis Records (PPASLR), University of Missouri, St. Louis.

Planned Parenthood Federation of America (I) Records, (PPFAR) Sophia Smith Collection, Smith College.

Planned Parenthood League of Detroit Records (PPLDR), 1932–79. Bentley Historical Library, University of Michigan, Ann Arbor.

Planned Parenthood League of Massachusetts Records (PPLMR), Sophia Smith Collection, Smith College.

Planned Parenthood of Western Pennsylvania Records (PPWPR), University of Pittsburgh Library.

Margaret Sanger Papers (MSP-C), Collected Documents Series, ed. Esther Katz (Bethesda, Md.: University Microfilms of America, 1996).

Margaret Sanger Papers (MSP-L), Library of Congress.

Margaret Sanger Papers (MSP-S), Sophia Smith Collection, Smith College (Bethesda, Md.: University Microfilms of America, 1995).

Margaret Sanger Papers, Unfilmed Portion (MS Unfilmed), Sophia Smith Collection, Smith College.

William Hazlett Upson Papers (Upson), Bailey Howe Library, University of Vermont (Burlington).

Gertrude Weil Papers (Weil), North Carolina State Archives.

ARTICLES AND MONOGRAPHS

ABCL. "Why Affiliate with the American Birth Control League?" May 1935 (MSP-L 28:61).

Alexander, W. G. "A Medical Viewpoint." *Birth Control Review* 16:6 (June 1932): 175.

Anderson, Maria H. "Private Choices vs. Public Voices: The History of Planned Parenthood in Houston." Rice University, Ph.D. diss., 1998.

Anonymous. "Clinic Reports: Birth Control Education Center." *JOC* 3:5 (May 1938): 68–71.Beisel, Nicola. *Imperiled Innocents: Anthony Comstock and Family Reproduction in Victorian America.* Princeton: Princeton University Press, 1997.

———. "Clinic Reports: Recreations Rooms and Settlement Birth Control Clinic, New York City." *JOC* 2:6–7 (June–July 1937): 164.

Beisel, Nicola. *Imperiled Innocents: Anthony Comstock and Family Reproduction in Victorian America.* Princeton: Princeton University Press, 1997.

Birth Control Clinical Research Bureau. *How to Establish a Birth Control Clinic.* New York: BCCRB, 1938.

Bocker, Dorothy. *Birth Control Methods.* New York: BCCRB, 1924.

Bousfield, Midian O. "Negro Public Health Work Needs Birth Control." *Birth Control Review* 16:6 (June 1932): 170.

Brodie, Janet Farrell. *Contraception and Abortion in 19th-Century America.* Ithaca, N.Y.: Cornell University Press, 1994.

Caron, Simone M. *Who Chooses? American Reproductive History since 1830.* Gainesville: University of Florida Press, 2008.

Chen, Constance. *The Sex Side of Life: Mary Ware Dennett's Pioneering Battle for Birth Control and Sex Education.* New York: New Press, 1996.

Chesler, Ellen. "Interview with Sarah Marcus." *Women's Studies Manuscript Collections from the Schlesinger Library, Radcliffe College. Series 3, Sexuality, Sex Education, and Reproductive Rights.* Bethesda, Md.: University Microfilms of America, 1994.

———. *Woman of Valor: Margaret Sanger and the Birth Control Movement in America.* New York: Simon and Schuster, 1993.

Condit, Jessie. "Underprivileged." *BCR* 10:4 (Apr. 1926): 115–17.

Cooper, George M., Frances Roberta Pratt, and Margaret J. Hapgood, "Four Years of Contraception as a Public Health Service in North Carolina." *American Journal of Public Health* 31:12 (Dec. 1941): 1248–52.

Dennett, Mary Ware. *Birth Control Laws: Shall We Keep Them or Abolish Them?* New York: Grafton Press, 1926.

Dickinson, Robert Latou, and Woodbridge Morris. "Birth Control Centers: A Report of 202 in the United States for the Year 1939." *Journal of the American Medical Association* 115 (1940): 591–93.

Dienes, C. Thomas. *Law, Politics, and Birth Control.* Urbana: University of Illinois Press, 1972.

Du Bois, W. E. B. "Black Folk and Birth Control." BCR 16:6 (June 1932): 166–67.

Fee, Elizabeth, "Public Health and the State: The United States." *The History of Public Health and the Modern State*, ed. Dorothy Porter. Atlanta: Rodopi, 1994. 224–75.

Ferebee, Dorothy. "Planned Parenthood as a Public Health Measure for the Negro Race." *Human Fertility* 7:1 (Feb. 1942): 7–10.

Fisher, Constance. "The Negro Social Worker Evaluates Birth Control." BCR 16:6 (June 1932): 174–75.

Franks, Angela. *Margaret Sanger's Eugenic Legacy: The Control of Female Fertility.* New York: McFarland, 2005.

Garrow, David J. *Liberty and Sexuality: The Right to Privacy and the Making of Roe V. Wade.* New York: Macmillan, 1994.

Gordon, Linda. *The Moral Property of Women: A History of Birth Control Politics in America.* Urbana: University of Illinois Press, 2002.

Granger, Isabella V. "Birth Control in Harlem." BCR 22:5 (May 1938): 91–92.

Guttmacher, Lenore, comp. *Planned Parenthood Beginnings: Affiliate Histories.* Houston: Margaret Sanger Centennial, 1979.

Hart, Henriette. "In the Homes of the Poor." BCR 10:12 (Dec. 1927): 319–20.

Hart, Jamie. "Who Should Have the Children? Discussions of Birth Control among African-American Intellectuals, 1920–1939." *Journal of Negro History* 79:1 (Winter 1994): 71–84.

Haslett, Diana C. "Hull House and the Birth Control Movement: An Untold Story." *Affilia: Journal of Women and Social Work* 12:3 (Fall 1997): 261–77.

Holz, Rosemarie Petra. "The Birth Control Clinic in America: Life Within, Life Without, 1923–1972." University of Illinois, Ph.D. diss., 2002.

———. "Nurse Gordon on Trial: Those Early Days of the Birth Control Clinic Movement Reconsidered." *Journal of Social History* 39:1 (Fall 2005): 112–40.

Johnson, Charles S. "A Question of Negro Health." *Birth Control Review* 16:6 (June 1932): 167–69.

Katz, Esther, ed., with Cathy Moran Hajo and Peter C. Engelman. *The Selected Papers of Margaret Sanger, Volume 1: The Woman Rebel, 1900–1928.* Urbana: University of Illinois Press, 2002.

———. *The Selected Papers of Margaret Sanger. Volume 2: Birth Control Comes of Age, 1928–1939.* Urbana: University of Illinois Press, 2007.

Kavinoky, Nadina R. "California Public Health and Mothers' Clinics." *Practice of*

Contraception, ed. Margaret Sanger and Hannah M. Stone. Baltimore: Williams & Wilkins, 1931. 205–8.

Kevles, Daniel. *In the Name of Eugenics: Genetics and the Uses of Human Heredity.* Cambridge: Harvard University Press, 1995.

Kopp, Marie E. *Birth Control in Practice.* Baltimore: Williams & Wilkins, 1931.

Ladd-Taylor, Molly. *Raising a Baby the Government Way: Mothers' Letters to the Children's Bureau, 1915–1932.* New Brunswick, N.J.: Rutgers University Press, 1986.

Lamport, Natalie. "Recreation Rooms and Settlement Birth Control" (MSP-L 32:276–94).

Leung, Marianne. "'Better Babies': The Arkansas Birth Control Movement during the 1930s." University of Memphis, Ph.D. diss., 1996.

Lewis, E. S., and N. Louise Young. "Baltimore's Negro Maternal Health Center: How It Was Organized." *BCR* 22:5 (May 1938): 94.

Lindemeyer, Kriste. "Expanding Birth Control to the Hinterlands: Cincinnati's First Contraceptive Clinic as a Case Study, 1929–1931." *Mid-America: An Historical Review* 77:2 (Spring–Summer 1995): 145–73.

Marsh, Charlotte Delafield. "Birth Control Centers in Settlements." *BCR* 16:5 (May 1932): 141–42.

Martin, George. "'Police Can't Stop Me' Says Margaret Sanger." *New York Call*, Oct. 22, 1916.

McCann, Carole R. *Birth Control Politics in the United States, 1916–1945.* Ithaca, N.Y.: Cornell University Press, 1994.

Meckel, Richard A. *Save the Babies: American Public Health Reform and the Prevention of Infant Mortality, 1850–1929.* Baltimore: Johns Hopkins University Press, 1990.

Meldrum, Marcia L. "'Simple Methods' and 'Determined Contraceptors': The Statistical Evaluation of Fertility Control, 1957–1968." *Bulletin of the History of Medicine* 70:2 (Summer 1996): 266–95.

Meyer, Jimmy E. W. *Any Friend of the Movement: Networking for Birth Control, 1920–1940.* Columbus: University of Ohio Press, 2004.

———. "Birth Control Policy, Practice, and Prohibition in the 1930s: The Maternal Health Association of Cleveland, Ohio." Case Western Reserve University, Ph.D. diss., 1993.

Mullan, Fitzhugh. *Plagues and Politics: The Story of the U.S. Public Health Service.* New York: Basic Books, 1989.

Nash, Carol K. "Planned Parenthood for New York Mothers." *BCR* 2:4 (April 1937): 128–29.

NCFLBC. *A New Day Dawns for Birth Control.* New York: NCFLBC, July 1937.

Norton, J. W. R. "A Health Department Birth Control Program." *American Journal of Public Health* 29:3 (Mar. 1939): 253–56.

Pasadena Hospital Clinic "Increasing Clinic Attendance." *National Clinic Courier* (Jan. 1936): 1–2.

Pearl, Raymond. "Contraception and Fertility in 2,000 Women." *Human Biology* 4:3 (Sept. 1932): 363–407.

———. "Fertility and Contraception in New York City." *JAMA* 108:17 (Apr. 24, 1937): 1385–90.

Planned Parenthood Clinic of Pittsburgh. *Changing Clientele of the Planned Parenthood Clinic of Pittsburgh, 1932–1947*. Pittsburgh: PPCP, 1949.

Pomeroy, John L., comp. *Public Health and the Private Medical Practitioner.* Los Angeles: Los Angeles County Health Office, 1932.

Pope, Fannie S. "The Story of Birth Control in Michigan, 1922–1942" (PPLDR).

PPFA. *Better Health for 13,000,000*. New York: PPFA, 1943.

Pringle, Henry. "What Do the Women of America Think About Birth Control?" *Ladies Home Journal* (Mar. 1938): 14.

Reed, James. *From Private Vice to Public Virtue: The Birth Control Movement and American Society since 1830*. New York: Basic Books, 1978.

———. "Interview with Elizabeth Arnold." *Women's Studies Manuscript Collections from the Schlesinger Library, Radcliffe College. Series 3, Sexuality, Sex Education, and Reproductive Rights*, Nov. 1974, reel 3.

Roberts, Dorothy. *Killing the Black Body: Race, Reproduction, and the Meaning of Liberty.* New York: Pantheon Books, 1997.

Robinson, Caroline Hadley. "How Shall We Start a Clinic?" *BCR* 16:5 (May 1932): 143–44.

———. *Seventy Birth Control Clinics: A Survey and Analysis Including the General Effects of Control on the Size and Quality of Population.* Baltimore: Williams & Wilkins, 1930.

Robishaw, Ruth. "A Study of 4,000 Patients Admitted for Contraceptive Practice and Treatment." *American Journal of Obstetrics and Gynecology* 31:3 (Mar. 1936): 426–34.

Rodrique, Jessie M. "The Afro-American Community and the Birth Control Movement, 1918–1942." University of Massachusetts, Ph.D. diss., 1991.

———. "The Black Community and the Birth Control Movement." *Unequal Sisters: A Multicultural Reader in U.S. Women's History*, ed. Vicki Ruiz and Ellen DuBois. New York: Routledge, 1990. 333–44.

Rothman, Sheila M. *Woman's Proper Place.* London: Basil Blackwell, 1984.

Sanger, Margaret. *Autobiography.* New York: W. W. Norton, 1938.

———. "Clinics, Courts, and Jails." *BCR* 2:4 (Apr. 1918): 3.

———. *Family Limitation.* New York: Rablelais Press, 1914.

———. *Happiness in Marriage.* New York: Brentano's, 1926.

———. *Motherhood in Bondage.* New York: Brentano's, 1928.

———. *My Fight for Birth Control.* New York: Farrar & Rinehardt, 1931.

———. "An Open Letter to Birth Control Centers in America." *JOC* 1:1 (Nov. 1935): 12.

———. *Pivot of Civilization*. New York: Brentano's, 1922.

———. "Status of Birth Control: 1938." *New Republic*, Apr. 20, 1938.

———. *Woman and the New Race.* New York: Brentano's, 1920.

———, and Hannah Stone, eds. *Practice of Contraception.* Baltimore: Williams & Wilkins, 1931.

Schoen, Johanna. *Choice and Coercion: Birth Control, Sterilization, and Abortion in Public Health and Welfare.* Chapel Hill: University of North Carolina, 2004.

Seibels, Robert. "The Integration of Pregnancy Spacing Into a State Maternal Welfare Program." BCFA Annual Meeting, Jan. 23, 1940 (PPFAR).

Stevens, Rosemary. *In Sickness and In Wealth: American Hospitals in the Twentieth Century.* New York: Basic Books, 1989.

Stix, Regine K., and Frank W. Notestein. *Controlled Fertility.* Baltimore: Williams & Wilkins, 1940.

Stone, Abraham, and Hannah M. Stone. *A Marriage Manual: A Practical Guidebook to Sex and Marriage.* New York: Simon and Schuster, 1935.

Stone, Hannah M. "Notes on a Roundtable Discussion." Conference on Contraceptive Research and Clinical Practice, Dec. 30, 1936 (MSP-L 29:499).

———. "The Massachusetts Raid." *JOC* 2:10 (Oct. 1937): 181.

Tasker, Cora. "The Mothers' Clinic." *Hospital Social Service* 14 (1926): 251–53.

Tone, Andrea. *Devices and Desires: A History of Contraceptives in America.* New York: Hill and Wang, 2001.

Trolander, Judith Ann. *Professionalism and Social Change: From the Settlement House Movement to Neighborhood Centers, 1886 to the Present.* New York: Columbia University Press, 1987.

Vreeland, Francis McClellan. "The Process of Reform with Especial Reference to Reform Groups in the Field of Population." University of Michigan, Ph.D. diss., 1929.

Warner, Marie. "Research Recommendations," Dec. 9, 1935 (MSP-L 32:234, 33:755A, and MSP-S 61:790).

Williams, Doone, and Greer Williams. *Every Child a Wanted Child: Clarence James Gamble, M.D., and His Work in the Birth Control Movement.* Boston: Harvard University Press, 1978.

Worchester, Daisy Lee Worthington. "Public Health and Private Doctors." *Survey-Graphic* 23:4 (Apr. 1934): 149–55, 202–4.

Yarros, Rachelle S. "Birth Control and Social Hygiene." *BCR* 6:7 (July 1924): 199–203.

Index

CATHY MORAN HAJO is an adjunct assistant professor in New York University's Archives and Public History Program and an associate editor of the Margaret Sanger Papers Project.

The University of Illinois Press
is a founding member of the
Association of American University Presses.

Composed in 10/13.5 Janson Text
with Electra display
by Celia Shapland
at the University of Illinois Press
Manufactured by Thomson-Shore, Inc.

University of Illinois Press
1325 South Oak Street
Champaign, IL 61820-6903
www.press.uillinois.edu